Manual of Wire Bend

MANUAL OF WIRE BENDING TECHNIQUES

Eiichiro Nakajima, DDS, DMSc
Private Practice
Tokyo, Japan

Quintessence Publishing Co, Inc

Chicago, Berlin, Tokyo, London, Paris, Milan, Barcelona,
Istanbul, São Paulo, New Delhi, Moscow, Prague, and Warsaw

Library of Congress Cataloging-in-Publication Data

Nakajima, Eiichiro.
  Manual of wire bending techniques / Eiichiro Nakajima.
      p. ; cm.
  ISBN 978-0-86715-495-5
  1. Orthodontic appliances--Design and construction. 2. Wire. 3. Bending.
I. Title.
  [DNLM: 1. Orthodontics, Corrective--methods--Atlases. 2. Orthodontic
Appliances--Atlases. 3. Orthodontic Wires--Atlases. WU 417 N163m 2010]
  RK527.N35 2010
  617.6'43--dc22
                          2010010905

©2010 Quintessence Publishing Co, Inc

Quintessence Publishing Co Inc
4350 Chandler Drive
Hanover Park, IL 60133
www.quintpub.com

Editor: Bryn Goates Grisham
Design: Gina Ruffolo
Production: Angelina Sanchez

Printed in China

Table of Contents

Preface

Many people believe that we are in the age of straight archwires and that wire bending is no longer necessary. However, the straight wire technique, in which a thin elastic straight wire is inserted and replaced by increasingly thicker wires, does not allow adjustments according to the unique skeletal morphology, dysfunction, tooth size, and dentition of each patient as well as the patient's age, sex, and wishes. If such adjustments are not necessary, treatment results should be the same in all cases, but this is not reality. Nevertheless, it is true that recent advances in wire properties have changed clinical techniques, and the development of wire with high resilience has reduced (but not eliminated) the necessity of bending.

Another consideration is bracket design. The force of wire is transmitted to the periodontal tissue and alveolar bone via the brackets attached to the teeth, and the morphology and size of brackets differ according to the developer of each technique and among manufacturers. Though each bracket has torque, angulation, in/out, and morphology based on its original design, it is strange that only one type is used for most techniques, without alteration for the unique needs of each patient. There are only some brackets in which angulation and torque differ depending on whether or not tooth extraction is included in the treatment plan. Setting the skeletal morphology and function of each patient aside, there should be at least some accommodation for different shapes and sizes of the crown and root. In manufacturing, original criteria used in the research and statistical calculation performed by the developers of each technique are used as the basis for the design of brackets. For example, some years ago, brackets marketed as being specially designed for Asian and Hispanic patients became commercially available but were developed based only on samples of Japanese, Korean, Chinese, and Mexican populations. One could reasonably question why these specific nationalities were selected and on what basis these ethnicities were combined.

If a retail store offered shoes or clothing in only one size, no one would shop there. This absurd situation is analogous to the current state of the orthodontic market. Bringing straight wires to market merely to increase sales represents a misplacement of priorities. There are many brackets and straight wire techniques based only on the morphologic statistics of specific population groups without consideration for biology or individual differences.

The author considers any bracket or wire acceptable if it is easy to use, prefers techniques that are as effective and efficient as possible, and uses only biologically compatible wires and brackets. Overly complicated wire bending is not necessary. This book was written with this perspective in mind and for the purpose of serving as a guide for good clinical practice.

CHAPTER 1

Mastering the Fourth-Order Bend

To say that success in orthodontic treatment is not dependent on individual wire bending techniques would undoubtedly draw criticism. Not only in orthodontics but also in any field that requires the use of specific techniques, such as implant dentistry, periodontal surgery, and oral surgery, the mastering of techniques themselves tends to be seen as the final goal. However, such techniques are meaningless without an understanding of to what and where they lead.

Orthodontic textbooks contain descriptions of first-, second-, and third-order bends. The first-order bend is in or out, the second-order bend is up or down, and the third-order bend is torque. These bends essentially relate to adapting wire on plaster casts. Casts are obtained by reproducing the very limited information provided by the teeth, gingiva, and palate at the time of impression taking. Casts do not contain information about the alveolar bone, periodontal membrane, gingiva, lingual frenum and corpuscles, or tongue. Wire bending based on limited information produces only correspondingly limited results.

Wire is used to apply force to a living organism. The teeth and dental arches are components of living organisms (ie, patients) and are part of the oral cavity, not lifeless objects separated from the individual.

Since the subjects of wire bending are living organisms, changes in these individuals cannot be discussed without reference to time. Time represents life stages from conception through birth, growth and development, and aging to death in each individual. Moreover, these individuals can live only in the environment of Earth. Humans developed the ability to walk on two legs as they evolved. The critical problem of how to balance the body in an upright position in the face of gravity had to be solved, and the morphology and function of various organs in the oral cavity evolved during this process. How can there be any meaning in aligning teeth and dental arches without considering this evolutionary process?

The fourth-order bend, therefore, is incorporating all the above-described factors into wire as information. Of course, it is impossible to incorporate all information into only one wire. One of the important purposes of clinical dentistry is to send signals to the brain via sensory organs distributed throughout the entire body, elicit appropriate orders from the brain to the muscles, and induce necessary and adequate muscle function. The fourth-order bend is a tool to achieve this. Thus, the fourth-order bend is information, rather than a method of bending.

CHAPTER 2

Trimming Casts

To appropriately position teeth in the jaws and improve masticatory function and esthetic appearance, three-dimensional custom casts trimmed according to the line of occlusion are necessary. When custom-made shoes are fabricated, wooden lasts (ie, three-dimensional casts of the feet) are made by hand or using a computer-aided design (CAD) system. Without these lasts, shoes perfectly fitting the feet of individuals cannot be made. Similarly, to create arches fitting the oral environment of individuals, custom casts are necessary (Fig 2-1). Of course, this process is easy using a CAD system, but the cast fabrication method described here is a less expensive method that can be readily performed by anyone.

Casts of arches with malocclusion are not simply cut with a trimmer. Each tooth is placed along its tooth axis, and the cast is cut along a plane that connects the mesial and distal contact points and is perpendicular to the tooth axis (Fig 2-2). A more accurate mesiodistal dimension can be obtained by measuring the mesial and distal contact points reproduced on this plane. In addition, the buccolingual dimension can be obtained by measuring the maximum protrusion areas on the buccal and lingual sides of each tooth, and the size of the offset or bayonet bend that should be given to the wire can also be estimated. If custom-made brackets could be obtained, brackets with in/out appropriate for each patient would be possible based on these values. At present, such brackets cannot be obtained, and the same brackets must be used even in the presence of marked differences in tooth width. These differences can be accommodated by bending the wire.

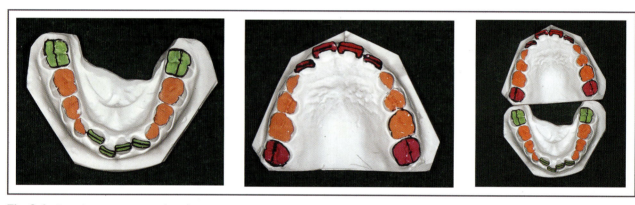

Fig 2-1 Custom casts trimmed at the contact points.

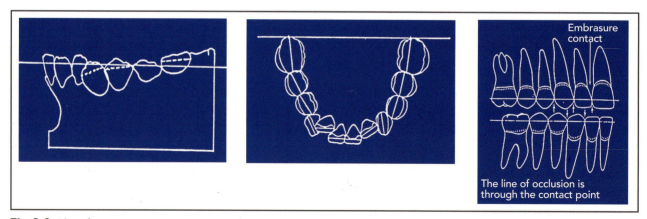

Fig 2-2 Plans for trimming a custom cast at the contact points.

CHAPTER 3

Basic Wire Bending

Selection of Pliers

In *The Book of Five Rings*, Miyamoto Musashi said that the highest attainment of the carpenter is that "his work is not warped," "the joints are not misaligned," and "the work is truly planed so that it meets well and is not merely finished in sections." To accomplish these goals, tools with various purposes have been developed. Musashi says that work that can survive over time is created by using these tools perfectly. It is ideal but impracticable to create tools suitable for each carpenter; therefore, to do good work, carpenters should put forth great effort to find the tools most suitable for them. The same is true with orthodontists.

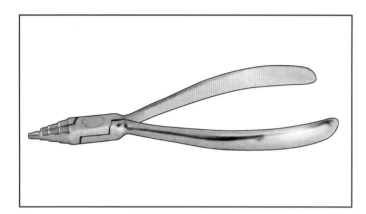

Fig 3-1 Biospecial pliers. These pliers are specially designed for use in bioprogressive therapy to bend 0.016 × 0.016 blue Elgiloy wire. They can also be used to bend other wires with similar properties.

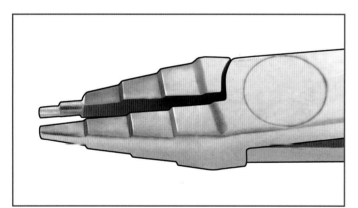

Fig 3-2 Biospecial pliers differ from other pliers in the beak structure. Both beaks are basically pyramidal in form, but the tip of one beak is modified into two tapering cylinders. The top and base of the first cylinder have diameters of 1.0 and 0.9 mm, respectively. The receiving beak contains a concavity at its tip that is equal to the diameter of the cylindric beak.

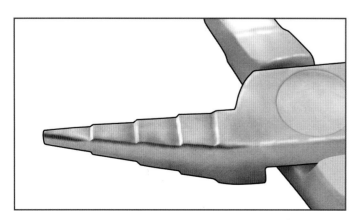

Fig 3-3 It is very important to bend wire at an exact spot. To aid in this task, there are four grooves on the beak of the biospecial pliers. These grooves correspond with widths of 3, 4, 5, and 6 mm. Use of these guides will provide desirable accuracy.

Fig 3-4 A view of the internal surface of the receiving beak shows a cylinder that is 2 mm wide the first 3.5 mm of its length. This allows the creation of a 90-degree bend at an exact 2-mm point. The bottom portion of the cylinder tapers to provide a gentle curve that is useful for adapting to canine curvature.

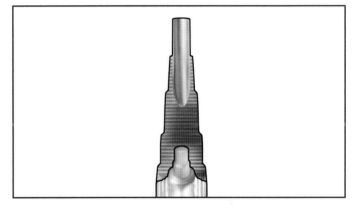

Fig 3-5 Joint portion of biospecial pliers. There is a 1-mm space at the junction of the two handles, which provides adequate spring action. Even when the pliers are gripped with excessive strength, this space reduces pressure on the beaks and thus prevents distortion. However, use of a gentle grip is always recommended.

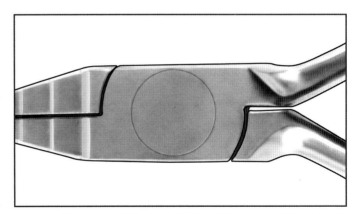

Fig 3-6 This top view of the biospecial pliers shows the cylindric beak and the semicircular receiving beak. The wire is inserted between the beaks, and the cylindric portion is used to form the loop. The ends of the pliers should not be used to bend thick wires with force.

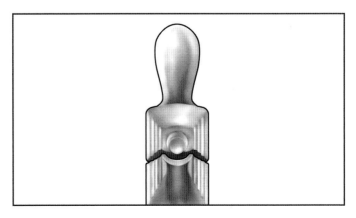

How to Hold Pliers

As warriors studying strategy repeatedly train themselves in the posture and way of holding swords and striking the enemy, orthodontists also should train themselves in the posture and way of holding pliers and using them to bend wire.

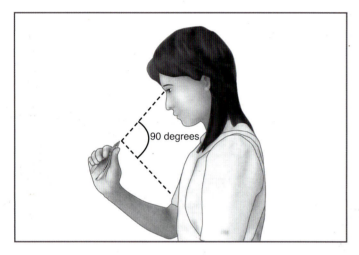

Fig 3-7 The pliers should be grasped gently with the right hand. A line from the eye to the end of the pliers should form a 90-degree angle with a line from the end of the pliers to the elbow.

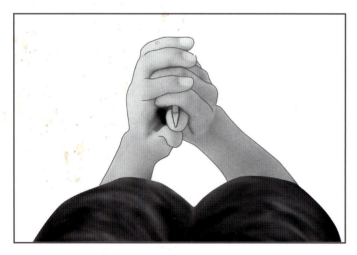

Fig 3-8 Place the left hand gently over the right hand. The thumb and index finger of the left hand should be able to move freely.

Wire Bending Procedures

The purpose of wire bending is to stimulate sensory organs in the teeth and periodontal tissues using the physical properties of wires to induce local changes in the periodontal tissue and alveolar bone and to activate necessary and adequate muscle function. For this, various methods are necessary; specific measurements such as 5 mm or 15 degrees is not applicable to all cases. The basic practice is shown in this section.

Vertical open loop

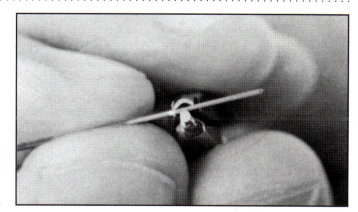

Fig 3-9 With the beaks facing toward you and the receiving beak above the cylindric beak, hold the wire at the first mark with the proximal end of the wire to the right.

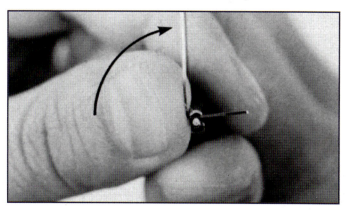

Fig 3-10 With the tip of the left thumb, bend the distal segment of the wire around the receiving beak 90 degrees.

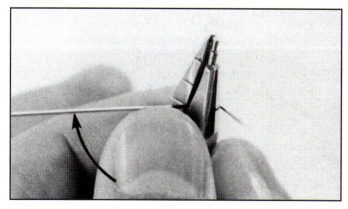

Fig 3-11 With the proximal end pointing down, hold the wire at the 6-mm (third) groove and bend the distal section 30 degrees.

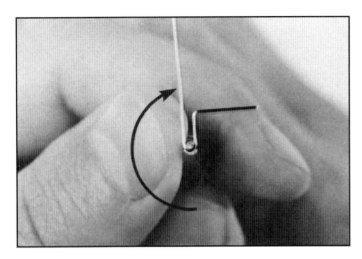

Fig 3-12 Hold the 30-degree angle symmetrically in the beaks with the cylindric beak on the concave side, and squeeze the handles firmly. Then complete the half loop with the left thumb.

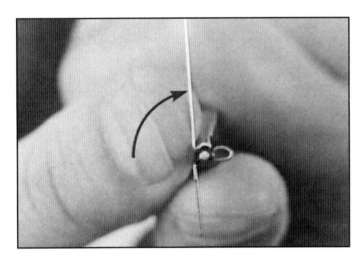

Fig 3-13 With the loop to the right, slide the receiving beak slightly to the right, and bend the distal segment 90 degrees to re-establish the standard line.

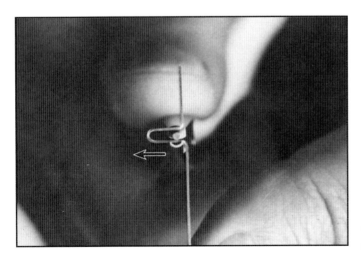

Fig 3-14 Failure to slide the receiving beak to the right will cause a distortion in the line.

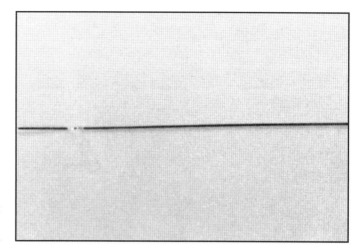

Fig 3-15 The wire should form a straight line when viewed from the top.

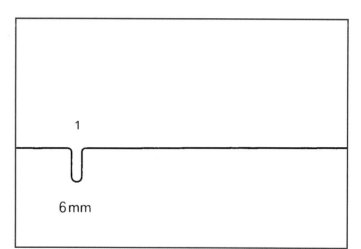

Fig 3-16 Check point 1. Place the loop over the diagram, and check its length, width, and shape.

Vertical helical closing loop

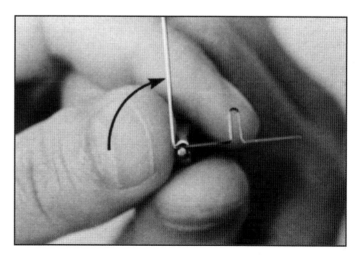

Fig 3-17 Hold the wire at the second mark. Bend the distal segment around the receiving beak 90 degrees in the same plane and direction as the previous loop.

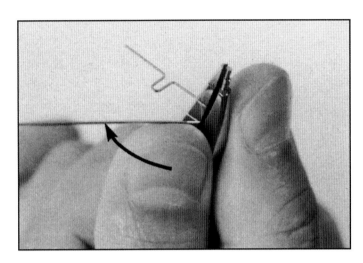

Fig 3-18 Hold the distal segment with the receiving beak in contact with the underside of the standard line at the 6-mm groove. Bend the wire 30 degrees toward the previous loop.

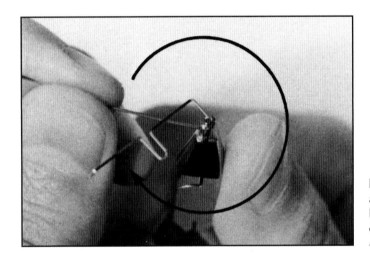

Fig 3-19 Make one and a half loops around the cylindric beak. Make sure to loop gradually toward the base of the cylindric beak in a clockwise direction.

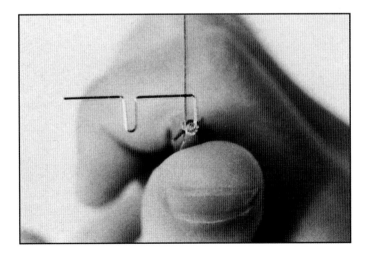

Fig 3-20 Bend until the two vertical legs become parallel.

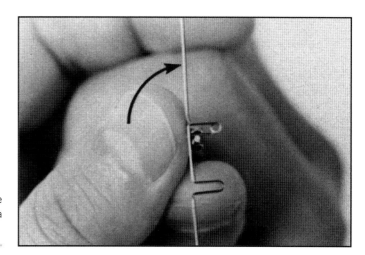

Fig 3-21 Hold the proximal leg of the loop, and bend it 90 degrees to form a straight line.

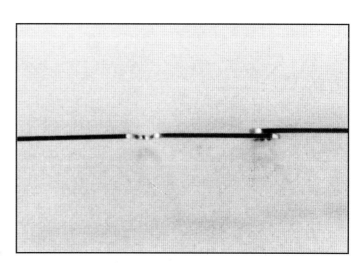

Fig 3-22 The top view of the wire should show no opening between the two vertical legs of the loop.

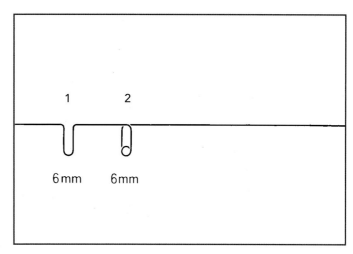

Fig 3-23 Check point 2. Align the wire with the diagram, and check the loop's length, width, and shape. Also check the accuracy of the distance between the two loops.

Horizontal "L" open boot loop

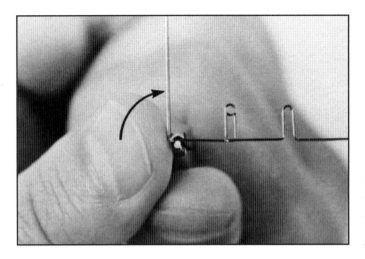

Fig 3-24 Hold the pliers on the third mark, and bend the wire 90 degrees in the same plane and direction as the other loops.

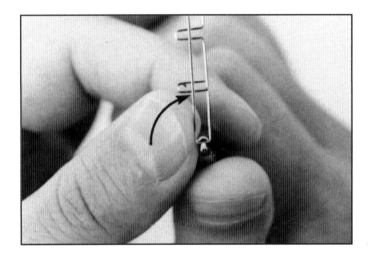

Fig 3-25 Hold the distal segment at the 3-mm groove, and bend it 90 degrees so that it is parallel with the standard line.

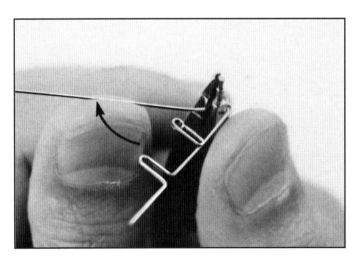

Fig 3-26 Hold the wire at the 4-mm groove, and bend it 30 degrees.

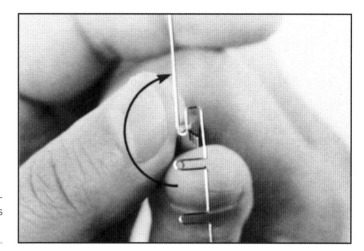

Fig 3-27 Place the wire around the cylinder to form a half loop so that the wire is parallel to the standard line.

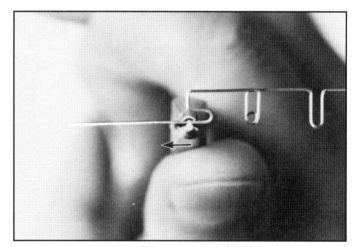

Fig 3-28 Move the receiving beak one wire width to the left of the vertical leg to ensure that the two vertical legs will be parallel.

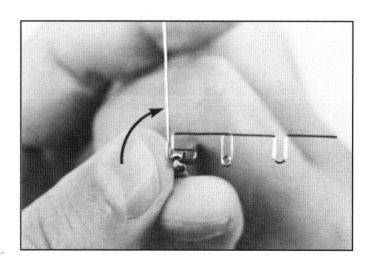

Fig 3-29 Bend the wire 90 degrees.

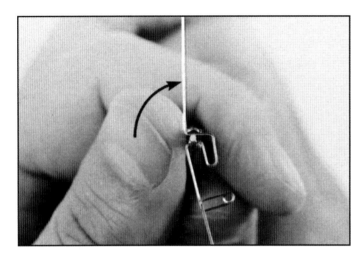

Fig 3-30 With the loop to the right, bend the distal wire 90 degrees so that it follows the standard line.

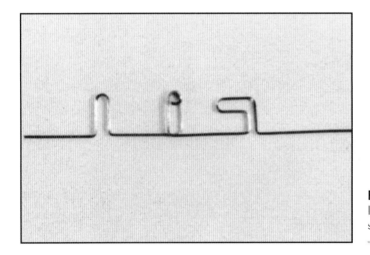

Fig 3-31 Even after forming the three loops, the standard line of the wire is straight.

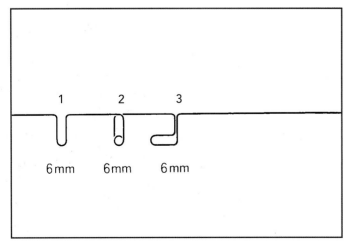

Fig 3-32 Check point 3. Align the wire over the diagram, and check the loop's length, width, and shape. Check for balance among the three loops.

Horizontal "T" open loop

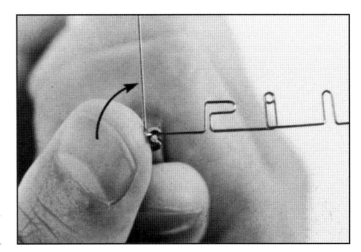

Fig 3-33 Hold the wire at the fourth mark, and bend the distal segment 90 degrees.

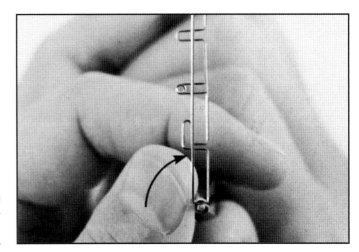

Fig 3-34 Hold the wire at the 3-mm groove, and bend it 90 degrees until it becomes parallel with the standard line.

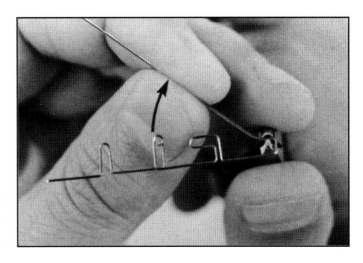

Fig 3-35 Use the first segment of the receiving beak to create a 30-degree bend away from the standard line in the distal segment.

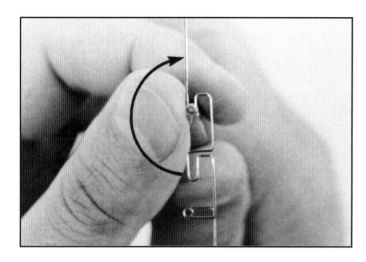

Fig 3-36 Form a half loop around the cylindric beak.

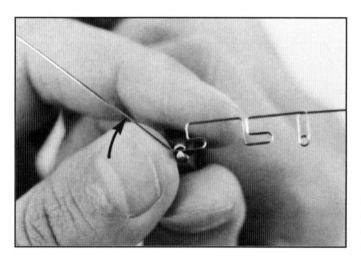

Fig 3-37 Slide the pliers 1 mm to the left of the vertical leg, and bend the wire 15 degrees.

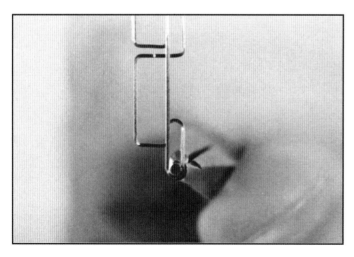

Fig 3-38 Form a half loop around the cylindric beak to overlap the previous half loop.

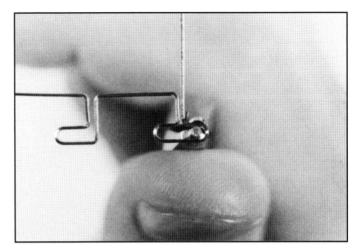

Fig 3-39 Use the tip of the receiving beak to make a 90-degree bend.

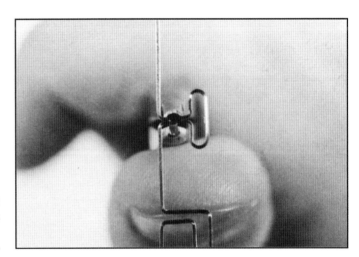

Fig 3-40 With the loop to the right, bend the distal segment of the wire 90 degrees to follow the standard line.

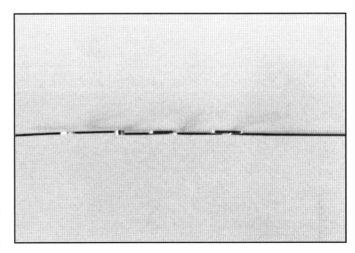

Fig 3-41 From the top, the wire appears to follow a straight line.

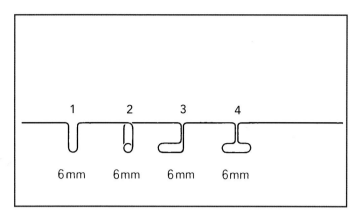

Fig 3-42 Check point 4. Align the wire over the diagram, and check the loop's length, width, and shape. Also check for symmetry.

Vertical approximated helical closing loop

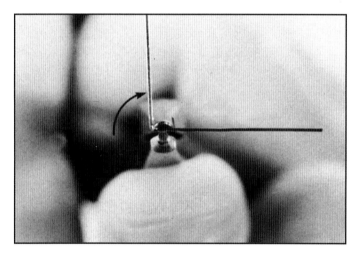

Fig 3-43 Hold the wire at the marked point, and bend it 90 degrees to an upright position.

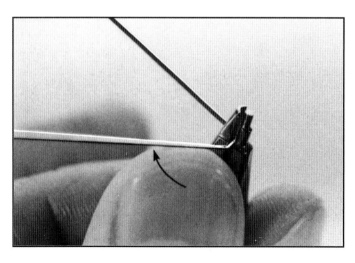

Fig 3-44 Hold the wire at the 3-mm groove, and bend it 30 degrees.

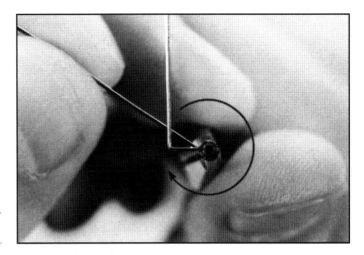

Fig 3-45 Wind the wire around the cylindric beak twice.

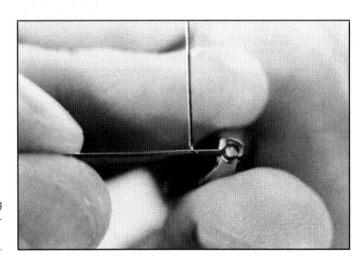

Fig 3-46 Use the edge of the receiving beak to bend the distal segment 30 degrees to align with the other vertical leg.

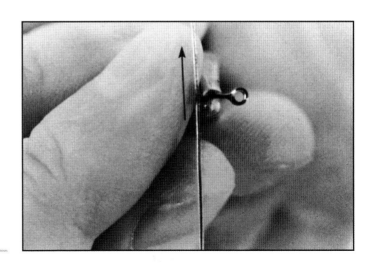

Fig 3-47 Bend to form a straight line.

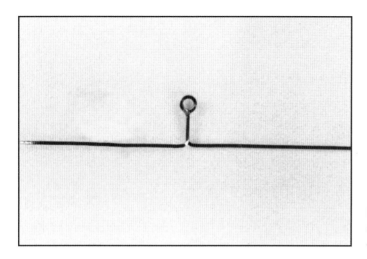

Fig 3-48 The vertical legs should overlap, and the wire line should be straight.

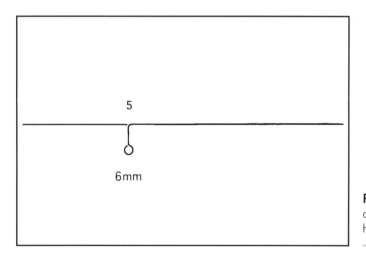

Fig 3-49 Check point 5. Align the wire over the diagram, and check the loop's height and balance.

Helical loop

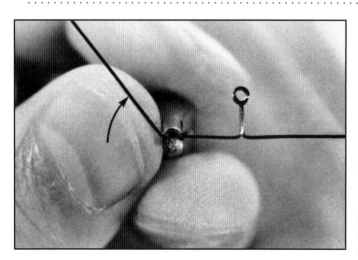

Fig 3-50 Hold the wire at the next marked point, and bend it 45 degrees.

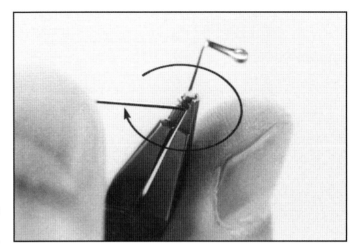

Fig 3-51 Make one and a half loops around the cylindric beak.

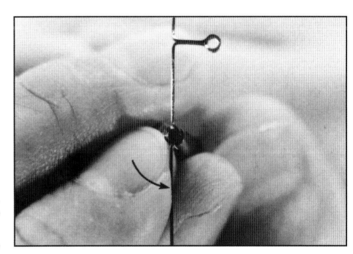

Fig 3-52 Bend the wire in the reverse direction so that it is positioned in the center of the loop.

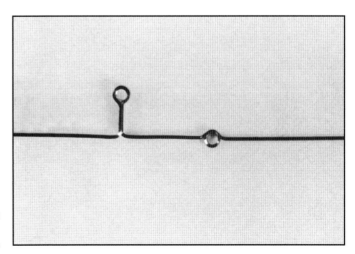

Fig 3-53 The standard line should be straight.

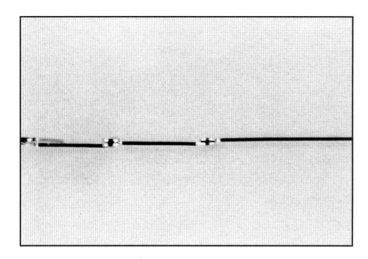

Fig 3-54 When viewed from the top, the standard line should deviate only the width of the loop.

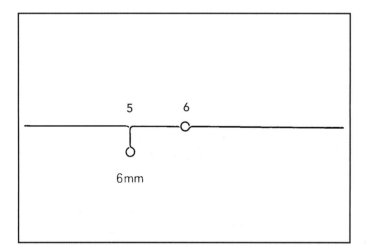

Fig 3-55 Check point 6. Align the wire over the diagram to confirm loop balance and the straightness of the standard line.

● Straight section (mandibular left)

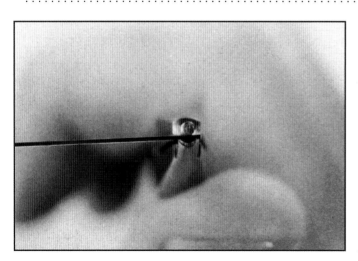

Fig 3-56 With the cylindric beak on top, hold the end of the wire in the tip of beaks.

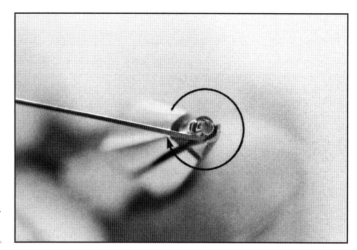

Fig 3-57 Make one loop around the cylindric beak, and form a stop loop.

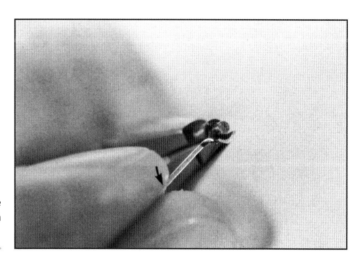

Fig 3-58 With the receiving beak at the point of contact, bend the wire around it in the opposite direction.

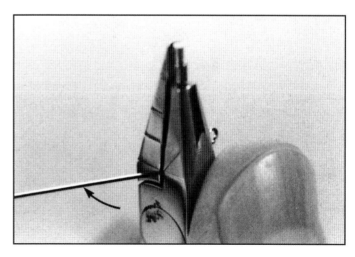

Fig 3-59 Make a 30-degree bend around the receiving beak, 8 mm posterior to the loop and perpendicular to the plane of the loop.

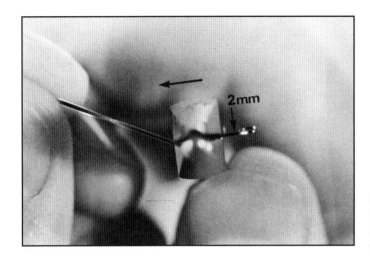

Fig 3-60 To measure this exact point, hold the wire at the 6-mm groove with the loop and 2 mm of wire protruding.

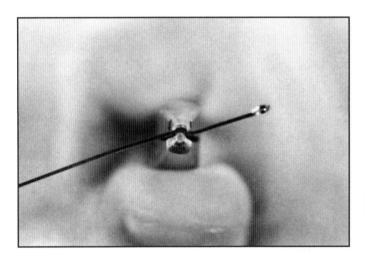

Fig 3-61 Place the edge of the receiving beak into the concavity of this bend, and squeeze to form an offset for the premolar.

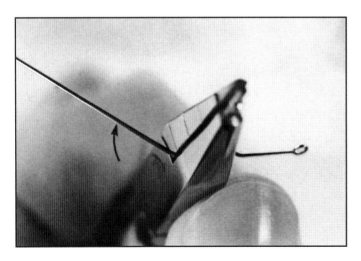

Fig 3-62 Make a 30-degree bend at 8 mm posterior to and in the same plane and direction as the previous offset.

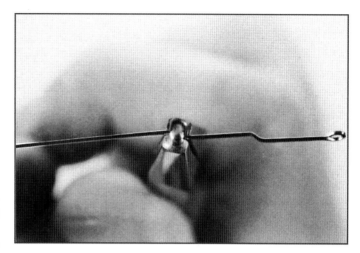

Fig 3-63 An offset for the molar is created using the second segment of the pliers.

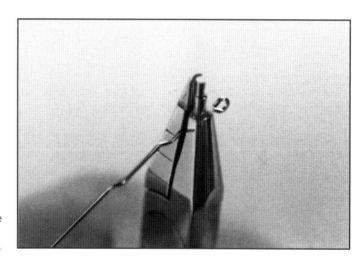

Fig 3-64 Form the canine curve using the contoured portion of the cylindric beak.

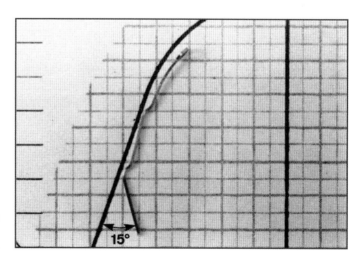

Fig 3-65 Form a 15-degree toe-in for the molar.

● Retraction section (maxillary left)

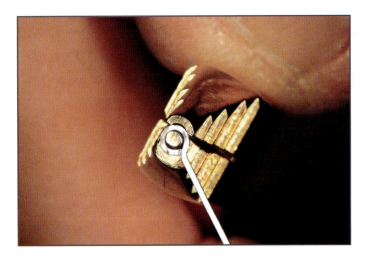

Fig 3-66 Make a stop loop.

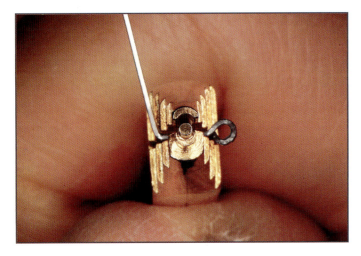

Fig 3-67 Hold the pliers pointing toward you with the cylindric beak on bottom, and bend the wire 90 degrees.

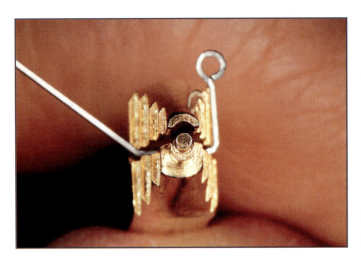

Fig 3-68 Place the wire at the 6-mm groove, and bend it 30 degrees anteriorly.

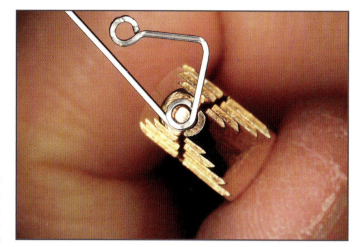

Fig 3-69 Make one and a half loops around the cylindric beak. Gradually loop toward the base of the cylindric beak in a clockwise direction. Avoid including torque.

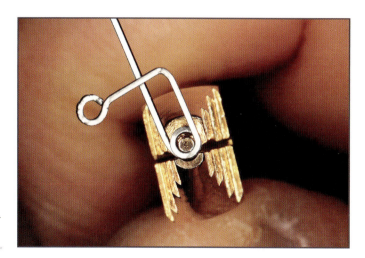

Fig 3-70 Bend the wire until the two vertical legs become parallel.

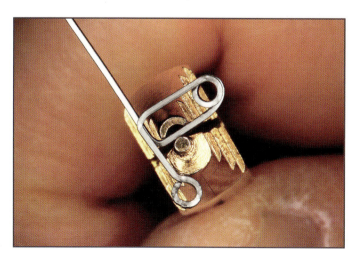

Fig 3-71 Slide the pliers one wire width to the right, and bend the distal end of the wire 90 degrees to follow the standard line.

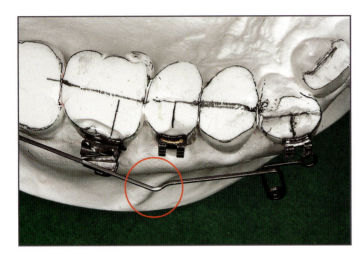

Fig 3-72 Mark the mesial wing of the second premolar, and add a bayonet bend (20 to 30 degree) using the second segment of the cylindric beak. Refer to the cast to determine the exact angle of the bend.

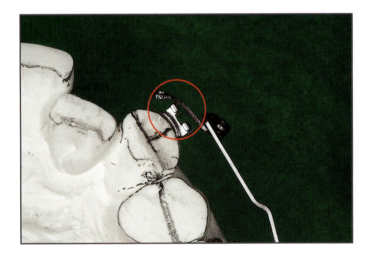

Fig 3-73 Curve the wire mesially from the maximum protrusion area of the canine bracket.

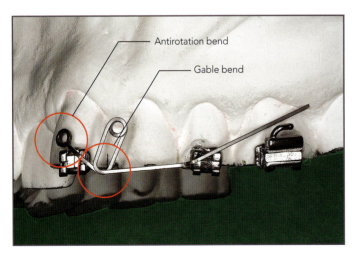

Antirotation bend

Gable bend

Fig 3-74 Adjust both legs of the vertical loop, and add a gable bend and an antirotation bend. The angles of these bends will differ depending on the specific case but are generally about 20 to 30 degrees.

Retraction section (mandibular left)

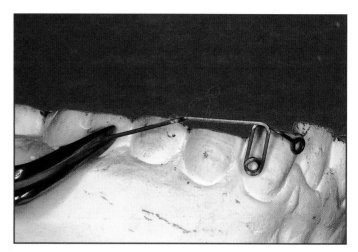

Fig 3-75 Refer to the maxillary left retraction section. The thickness and angle of each bend is determined based on the pretreatment cast.

Stabilizing helical section (maxillary left)

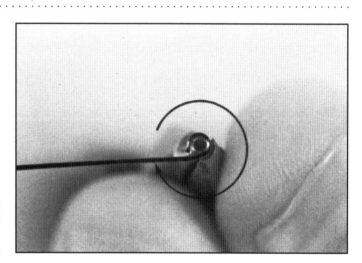

Fig 3-76 Hold the pliers pointing toward you, with the cylindric beak above the receiving beak, and form a loop anteriorly.

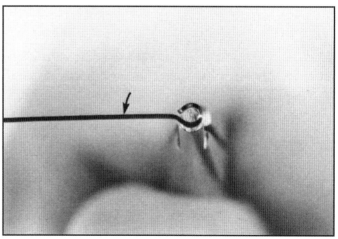

Fig 3-77 Without changing the position of the pliers, bend the wire 15 degrees in the reverse direction.

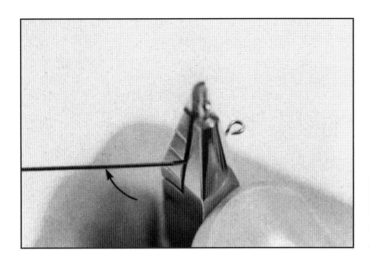

Fig 3-78 Use the groove on the receiving beak to make a 30-degree bend gingivally in the same plane as, and 8 mm away from, the loop.

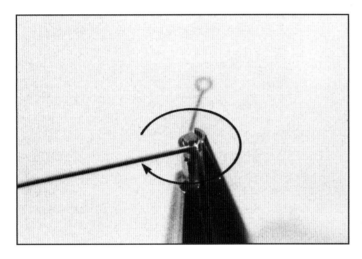

Fig 3-79 Form one and a half loops, avoiding the incorporation of torque.

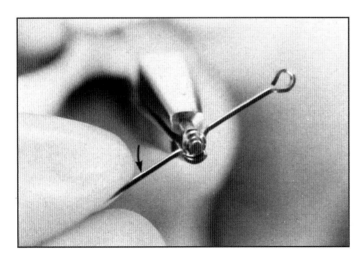

Fig 3-80 With the cylindric beak inside the loops, bend the wire 30 degrees in a reverse direction to straighten it.

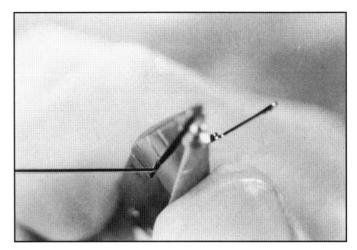

Fig 3-81 Hold the wire 3 mm anterior to the buccal tube mark. Bend the posterior segment 30 degrees buccally and perpendicular to the plane of the loops.

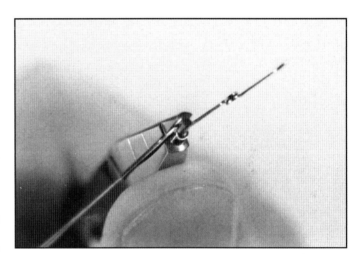

Fig 3-82 Form a molar offset using the second segment of the cylindric beak.

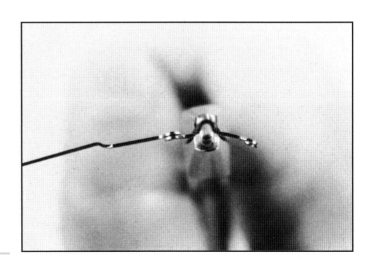

Fig 3-83 Bend the canine curve.

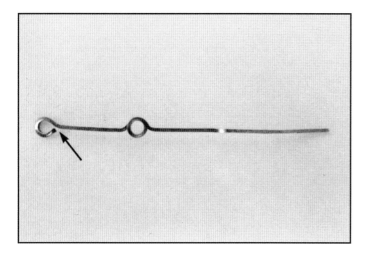

Fig 3-84 The open end of the stop loop should face gingivally.

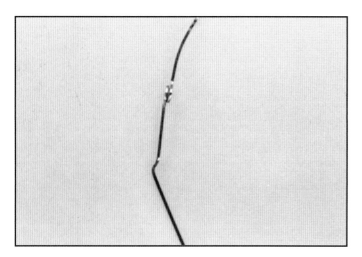

Fig 3-85 Top view shows that the helical loop is on the buccal aspect.

Mandibular utility arch

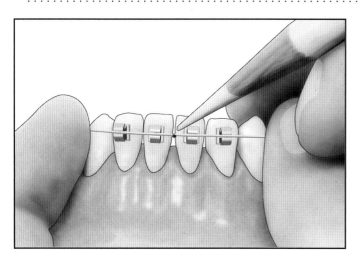

Fig 3-86 Align the central red mark of the preformed archwire with the contact point between the mandibular central incisors.

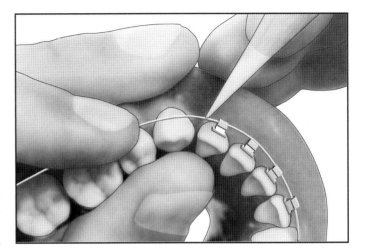

Fig 3-87 Mark the wire 1.5 mm distal to the bracket of the mandibular left lateral incisor.

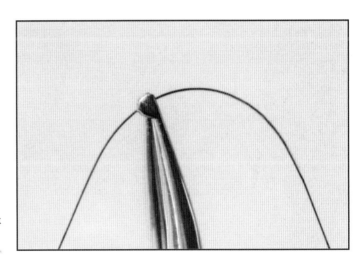

Fig 3-88 Hold the wire mesial to the mark with the tips of Howe pliers.

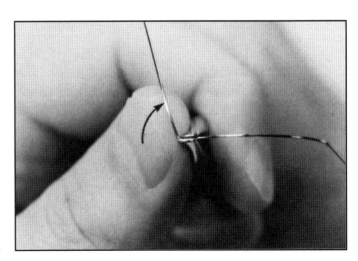

Fig 3-89 Bend the wire 75 degrees gingivally.

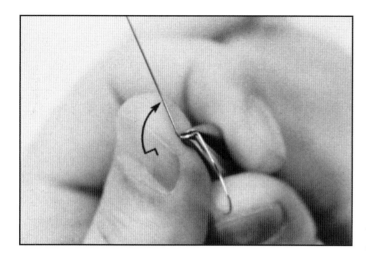

Fig 3-90 Using the Howe pliers, form an anterior step that has the same width as its tip.

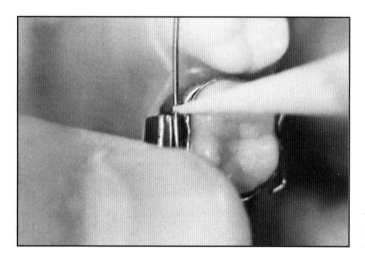

Fig 3-91 With the central red mark aligned with the midline, mark the wire at the mesial aspect of the buccal tube.

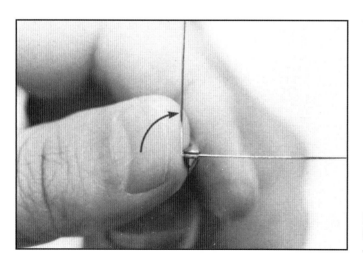

Fig 3-92 Hold the pliers at the mark, and bend the wire 90 degrees occlusally.

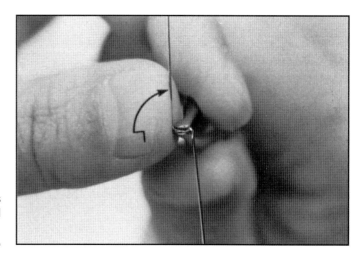

Fig 3-93 Use the width of the Howe pliers to bend the wire 90 degrees to the distal and parallel to the buccal bridge.

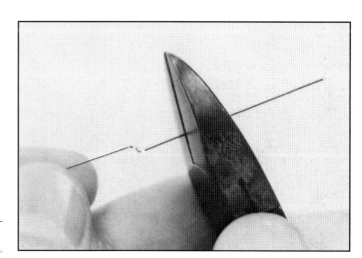

Fig 3-94 Cut the wire 9 mm from the posterior vertical step.

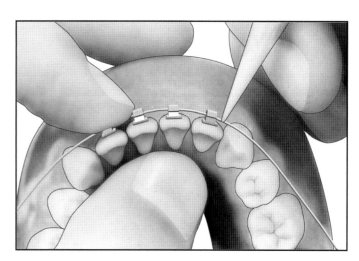

Fig 3-95 With the central red mark aligned with the midline, mark the wire 1.5 mm distal to the mandibular right incisor bracket.

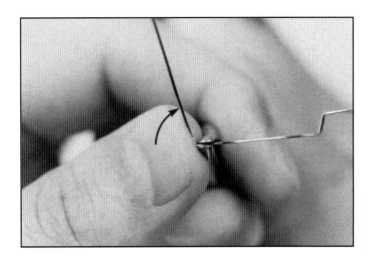

Fig 3-96 Hold the wire with the pliers mesial to this mark, and bend it 75 degrees gingivally.

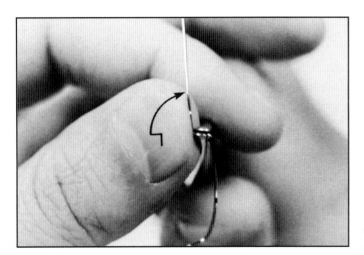

Fig 3-97 Form an anterior step the same width as the top of the Howe pliers.

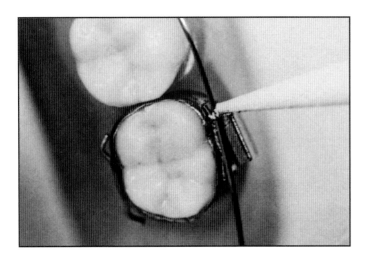

Fig 3-98 With the central mark aligned, mark the wire at the mesial aspect of the buccal tube.

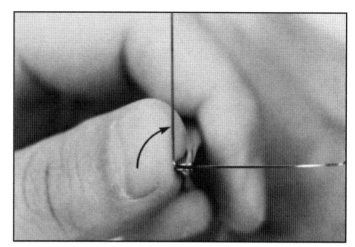

Fig 3-99 Hold the pliers on this mark, and bend the wire 90 degrees occlusally.

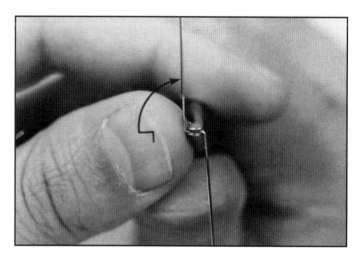

Fig 3-100 Use the width of the Howe pliers to bend the wire 90 degrees to the distal and parallel to the buccal bridge.

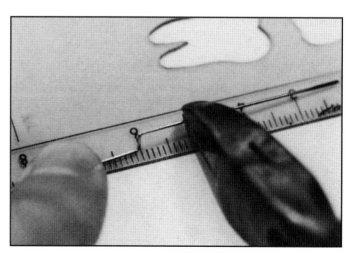

Fig 3-101 Cut the wire 9 mm from the posterior vertical step.

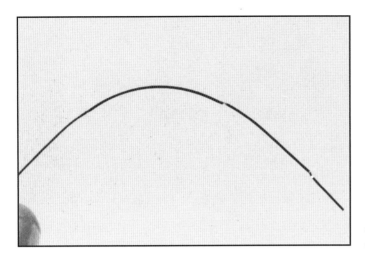

Fig 3-102 Check the symmetry at this stage.

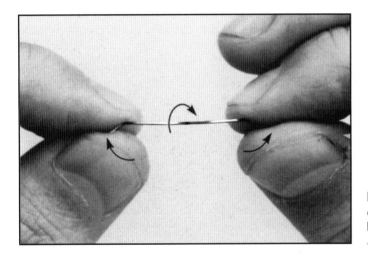

Fig 3-103 Incorporate lingual crown torque in the anterior segment. Flare out the buccal aspect during this procedure.

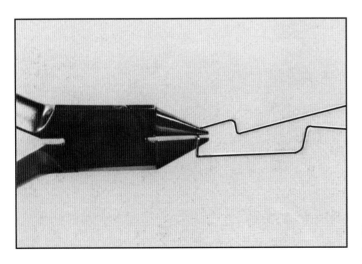

Fig 3-104 Check the amount of torque.

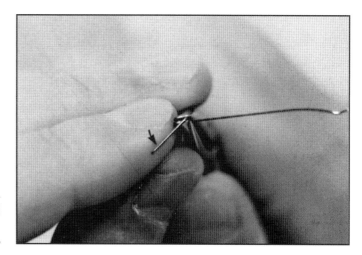

Fig 3-105 Give the left posterior segment a 30-degree toe-in at the vertical step.

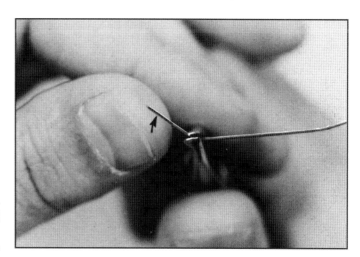

Fig 3-106 Give the right posterior segment a 30-degree toe-in at the vertical step.

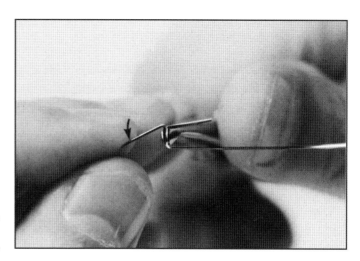

Fig 3-107 Place a 30-degree tip-back on the left posterior segment.

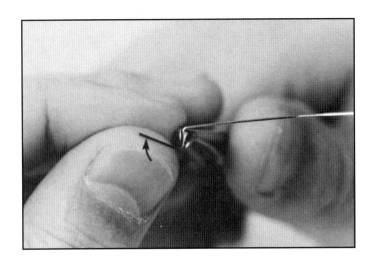

Fig 3-108 Place a 30-degree tip-back on the right posterior segment.

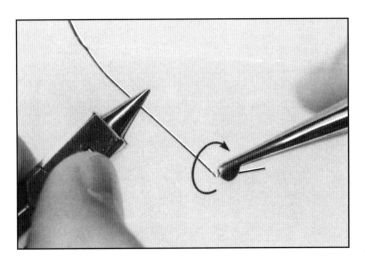

Fig 3-109 Place buccal root torque in the left posterior segment.

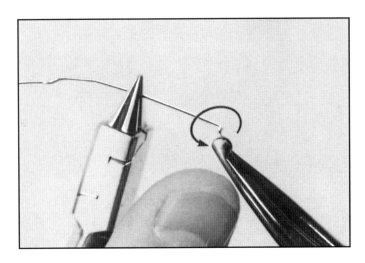

Fig 3-110 Place a similar amount of torque in the right posterior segment.

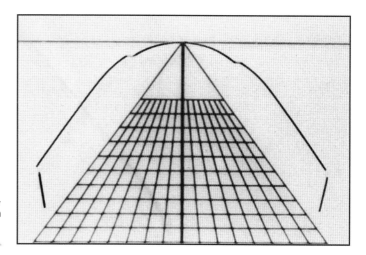

Fig 3-111 Increase the anterior curvature, and maintain the appropriate arch width posteriorly.

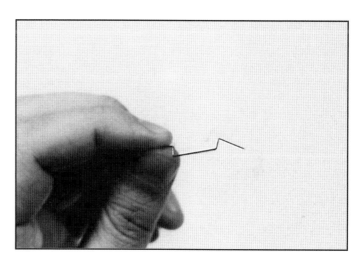

Fig 3-112 Check the posterior segments for uniformity between the left and right sides.

Maxillary closing utility arch

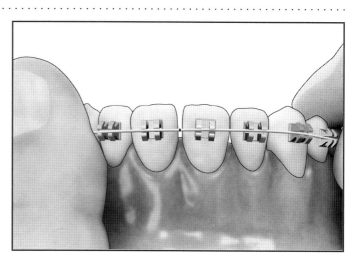

Fig 3-113 Align the central mark in the wire with the contact point between the two central incisors.

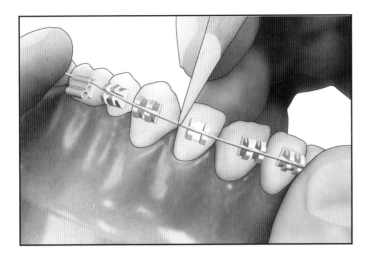

Fig 3-114 Mark the wire 2 mm distal to the maxillary left lateral incisor bracket.

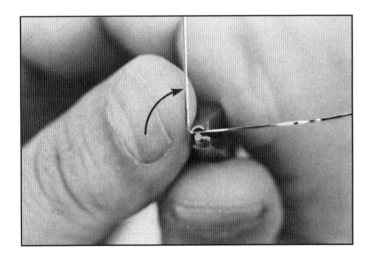

Fig 3-115 At this mark, bend the wire 90 degrees occlusally to form an anterior vertical step.

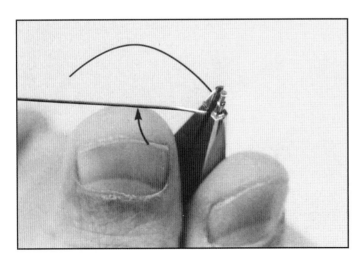

Fig 3-116 Align the last bend with the 3-mm groove, and bend it 30 degrees mesially.

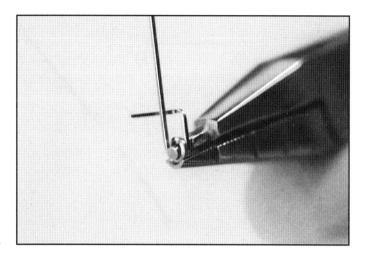

Fig 3-117 Form one and a half loops anterior to the step.

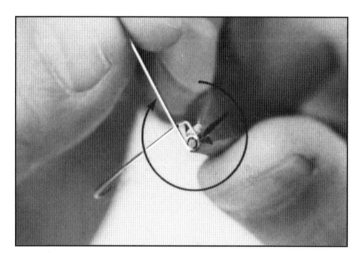

Fig 3-118 The loops should be outside the anterior segment.

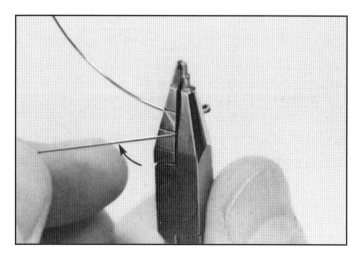

Fig 3-119 With the pliers against the gingival side of the anterior segment, align the wire with the 5-mm groove, and bend the vertical leg 30 degrees mesially.

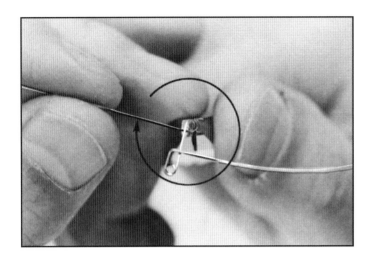

Fig 3-120 Using the cylindric beak as an axis, make a three-quarter loop anterior to and outside of the long vertical leg. The wire is now parallel with the standard line.

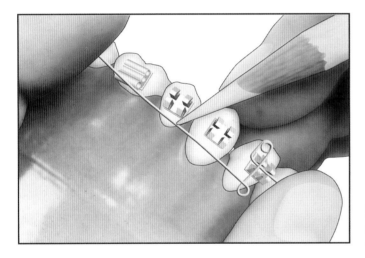

Fig 3-121 Mark the wire at the medial wing of the premolar bracket.

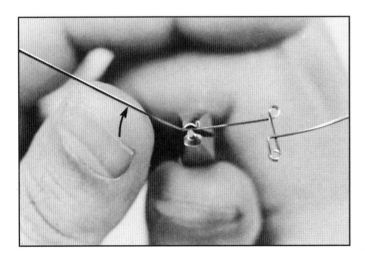

Fig 3-122 Position the receiving beak just mesial to the mark, and bend the wire 30 degrees gingivally.

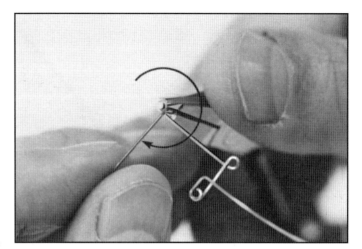

Fig 3-123 Using the cylindric beak as an axis, form a three-quarter loop distal to and outside of the resulting vertical segment.

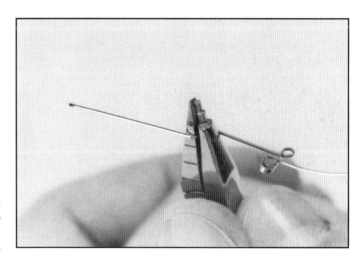

Fig 3-124 Align the wire with the 4-mm groove, and bend it 90 degrees distally to form a vertical step.

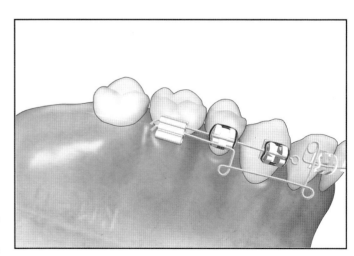

Fig 3-125 Cut the wire 3 mm distal to the end of the buccal tube.

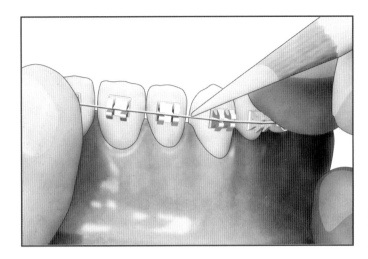

Fig 3-126 Mark the wire 2 mm distal to the maxillary right lateral incisor bracket.

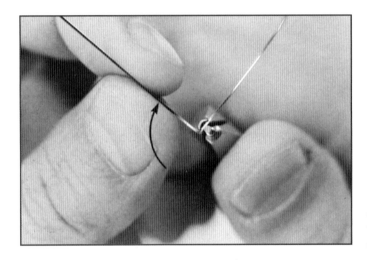

Fig 3-127 At this mark, bend the wire 90 degrees occlusally to form an anterior vertical step.

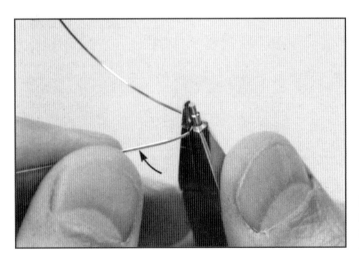

Fig 3-128 Align the last bend with the 3-mm line, and bend the wire 30 degrees mesially.

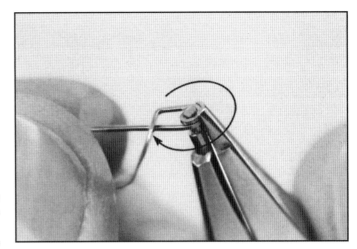

Fig 3-129 Continue to bend the wire around the cylindric beak, and make one and a half loops anterior to the step.

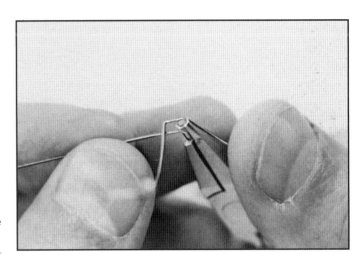

Fig 3-130 The loops should be outside the anterior segment.

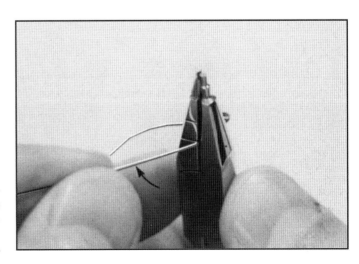

Fig 3-131 With the pliers against the gingival side of the anterior segment, align the wire with the 5-mm line, and bend the vertical leg 30 degrees.

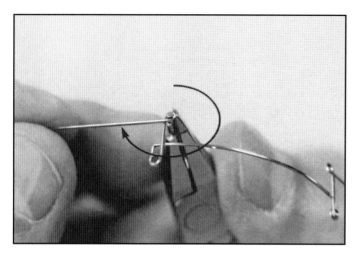

Fig 3-132 Using the cylindric beak as an axis, make a three-quarter loop anterior to and outside of the long vertical leg. The wire is now parallel with the standard line.

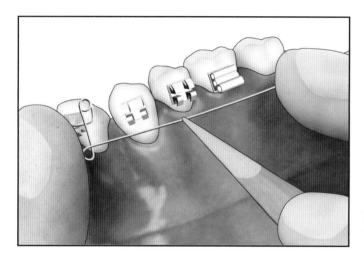

Fig 3-133 Mark the wire at the mesial wing of the first premolar bracket.

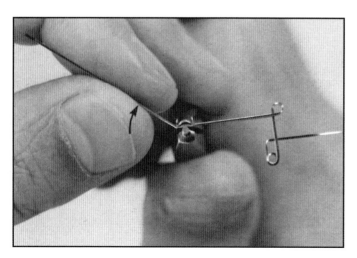

Fig 3-134 Position the receiving beak on the mark, and bend the wire 30 degrees gingivally.

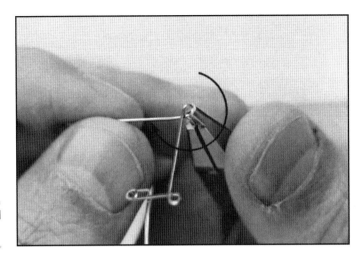

Fig 3-135 Using the cylindric beak as an axis, form a three-quarter loop distal to and outside of the resulting vertical segment.

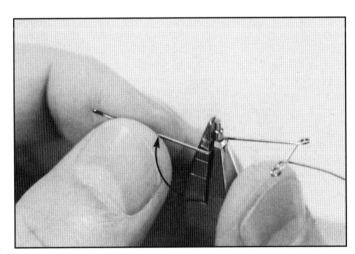

Fig 3-136 Position the wire at the 4-mm line, and bend it 90 degrees distally to form a vertical step and restore the standard line.

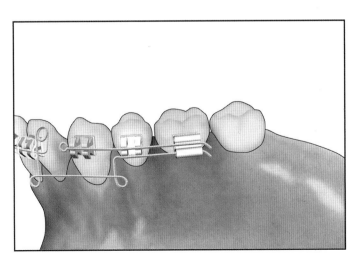

Fig 3-137 Cut the wire 3 mm distal to the end of the buccal tube.

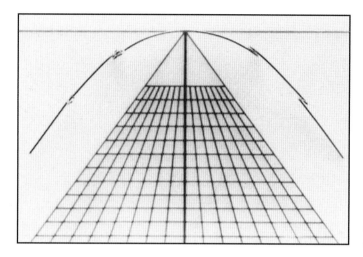

Fig 3-138 The wire should have considerable expansion at this stage.

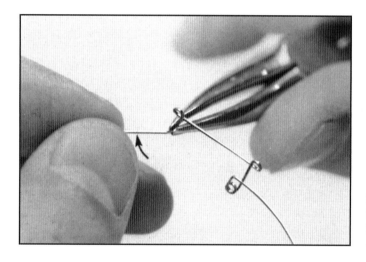

Fig 3-139 Add a toe-in while bending the left posterior vertical step with the Howe pliers.

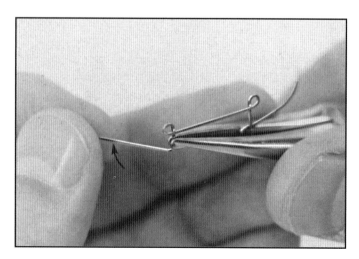

Fig 3-140 Add a toe-in to the right side in the same manner.

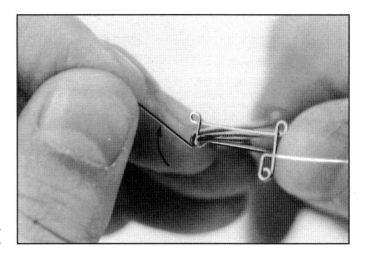

Fig 3-141 Add a tip-back to the left side.

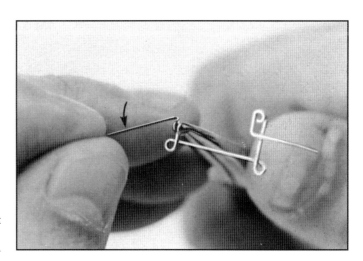

Fig 3-142 Add a tip-back to the right side.

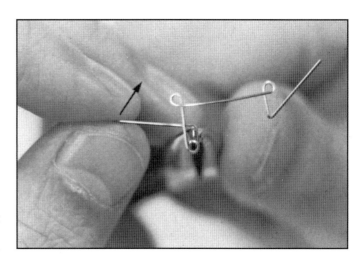

Fig 3-143 Increase torque by enlarging the angle between the anterior segment and the vertical leg of the left anterior step.

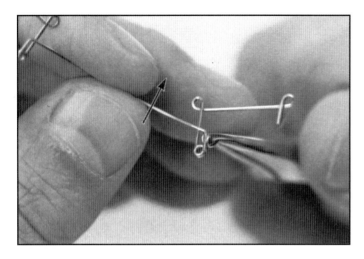

Fig 3-144 Repeat the previous procedure on the right side.

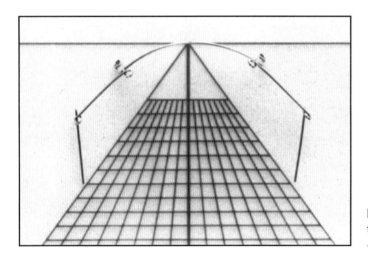

Fig 3-145 Adjust the toe-in, tip-back, and torque, and check for symmetry.

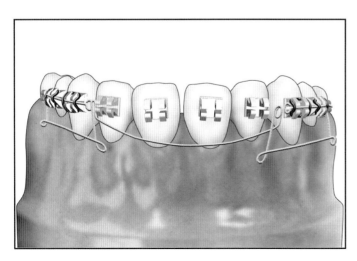

Fig 3-146 Insert the wire in the middle of the triple tube, and check for the amount of torque.

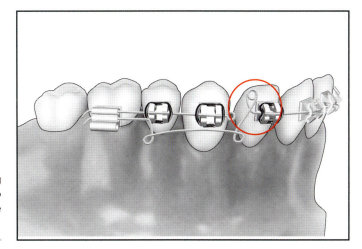

Fig 3-147 Activate the wire by cinching back distal to the left buccal tube. The two vertical legs of the anterior loops should be crossed.

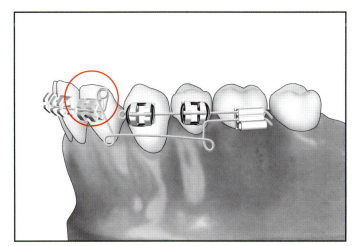

Fig 3-148 In the same manner, activate the right side. Cut the wire 3 mm distal to the end of the buccal line.

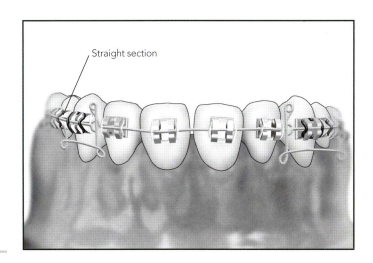

Straight section

Fig 3-149 Anterior view.

Mandibular ideal arch: Second premolar to second premolar (.016 × .022 wire)

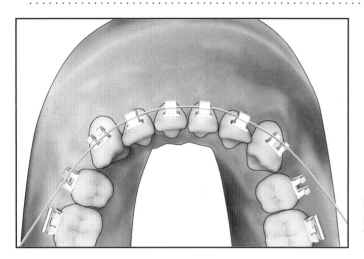

Fig 3-150 Position the central red mark at the contact point between the two central incisors.

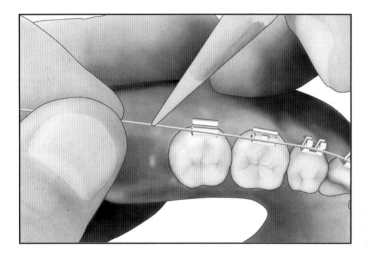

Fig 3-151 Mark and cut the wire 5 mm distal to the left buccal tube.

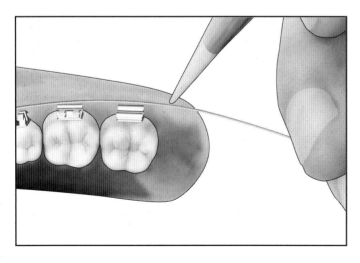

Fig 3-152 Mark and cut the wire 5 mm distal to the right buccal tube.

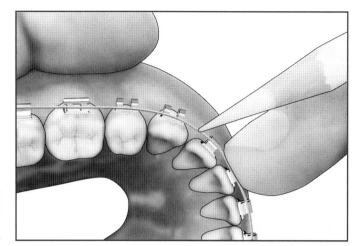

Fig 3-153 Mark the wire at the contact point between the left lateral incisor and canine.

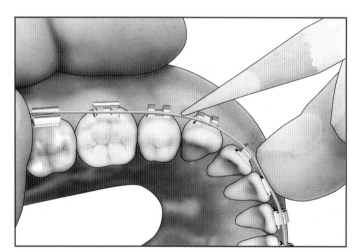

Fig 3-154 Mark the wire at the contact point between the left canine and premolar.

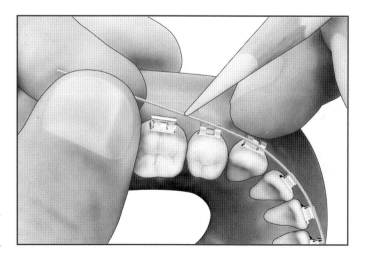

Fig 3-155 Mark the wire 2 mm mesial to the left buccal tube.

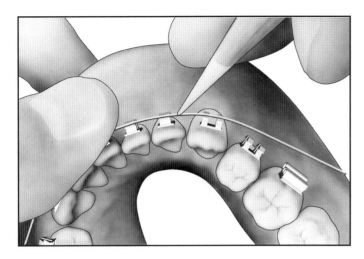

Fig 3-156 Mark the wire over the contact point between the right lateral incisor and canine.

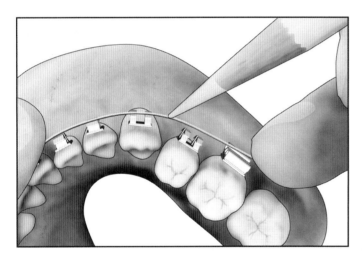

Fig 3-157 Mark the wire over the contact point between the right canine and premolar.

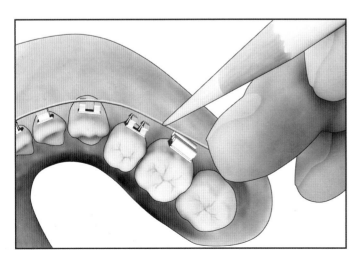

Fig 3-158 Mark the wire 2 mm mesial to the right buccal tube.

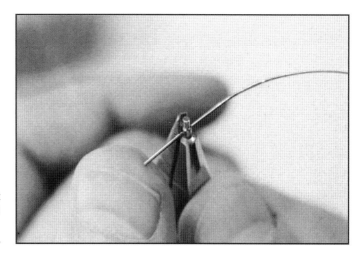

Fig 3-159 Mark the offset for the left molar. Grip the molar mark with the second segment of the cylindric beak.

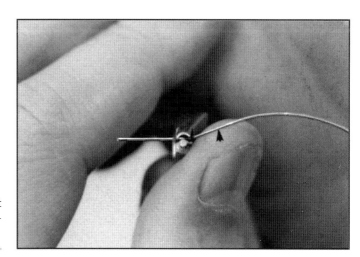

Fig 3-160 Bend the anterior segment around the receiving beak 15 degrees buccally with the left thumb.

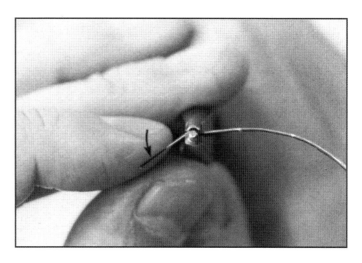

Fig 3-161 Bend the posterior segment 30 degrees lingually with the left index finger.

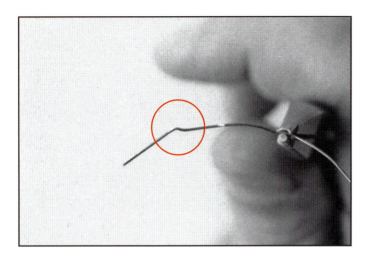

Fig 3-162 The bayonet bend for the left molar has been completed.

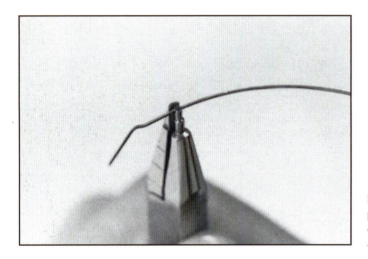

Fig 3-163 Grip the mark between the premolar and canine with the first segment of the cylindric beak.

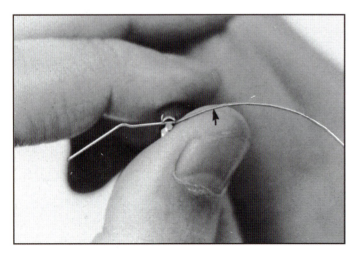

Fig 3-164 Bend the anterior segment around the receiving beak 15 degrees buccally with the left thumb.

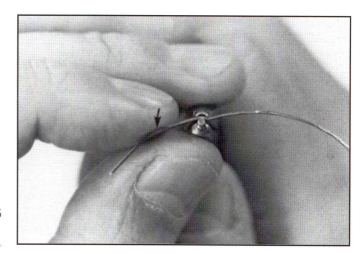

Fig 3-165 Bend the posterior segment 15 degrees lingually with the left index finger.

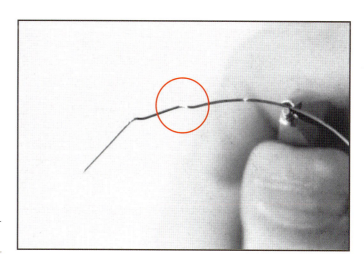

Fig 3-166 The mesial offset of the premolar has been completed.

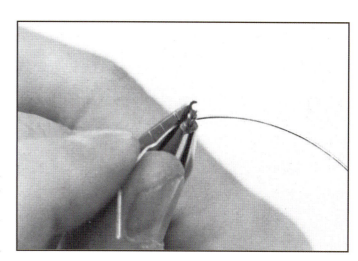

Fig 3-167 Grip the mark on the wire between the left lateral incisor and canine with the contoured portion of the pliers, and slide the pliers distally two or three times.

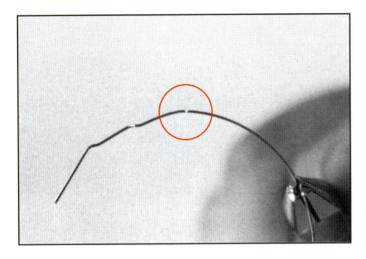

Fig 3-168 The left canine curvature has been completed.

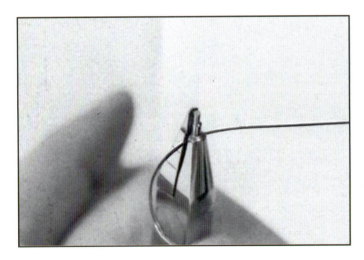

Fig 3-169 Grip the mark on the wire between the right lateral incisor and canine with the contoured portion of the pliers, and slide the pliers distally two or three times.

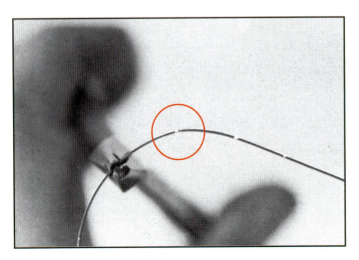

Fig 3-170 The right canine curvature has been completed.

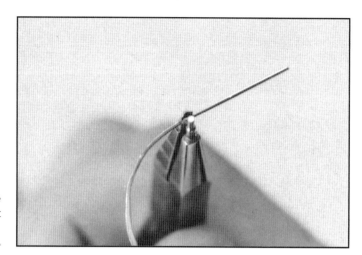

Fig 3-171 Grip the mark between the premolar and canine with the first segment of the cylindric beak.

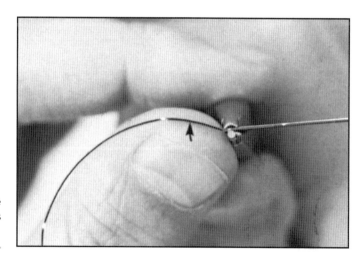

Fig 3-172 With the left thumb, bend the anterior segment of the wire 15 degrees buccally around the receiving beak.

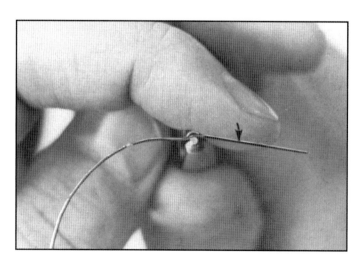

Fig 3-173 With the left index finger, bend the posterior segment 15 degrees lingually.

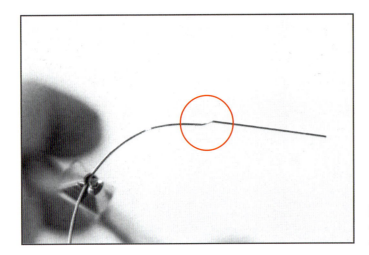

Fig 3-174 The premolar offset has been completed.

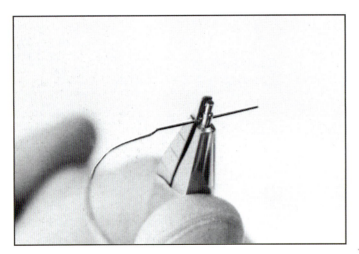

Fig 3-175 Grip the mark on the wire mesial to the right molar with the second segment of the cylindric beak.

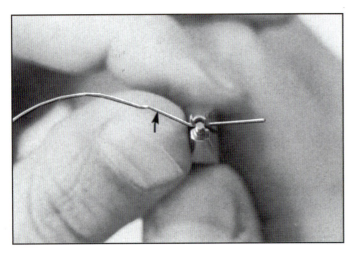

Fig 3-176 Bend the anterior segment 15 degrees buccally with the left thumb.

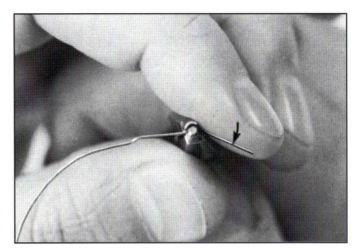

Fig 3-177 Bend the posterior segment 30 degrees lingually using the index finger.

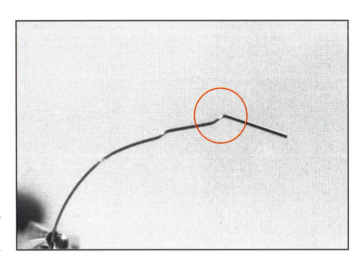

Fig 3-178 The bayonet bend in the molar area has been completed.

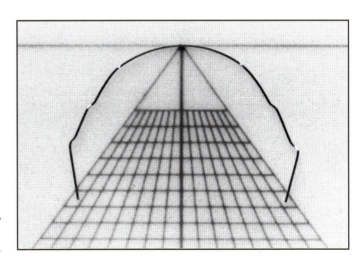

Fig 3-179 Complete the procedure by checking the arch form and symmetry.

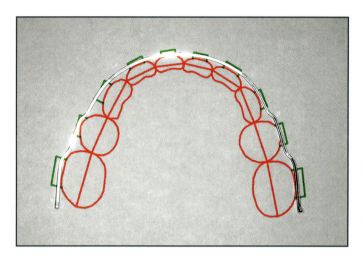

Fig 3-180 Check the thickness of the offset and bayonet bends as well as the symmetry of the arch according to the pretreatment mandibular visual treatment objective (VTO).

● Mandibular ideal arch: First molar to first molar (.016 × .022 wire)

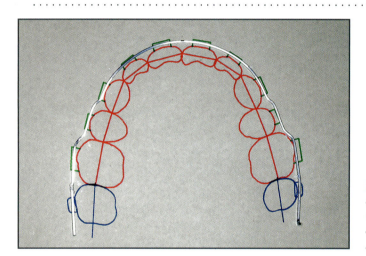

Fig 3-181 Mark on the wire the mesial contact points of the left and right second molars, and curve the wire slightly in the distal direction.

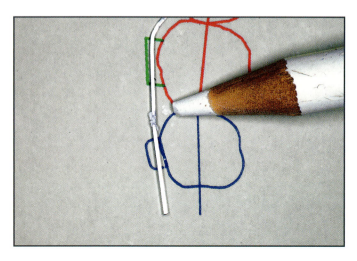

Fig 3-182 Referring to the mandibular VTO produced from the cast, curve the wire distally from the contact points, taking into consideration the difference in buccolingual crown width between the premolars and molars.

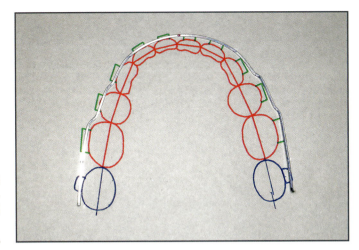

Fig 3-183 Mark on the wire the mesial contact points of the left and right first molars, and curve the wire slightly in the distal direction.

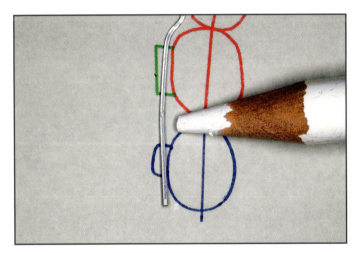

Fig 3-184 Referring to the mandibular VTO, curve the wire slightly in the distal direction from the contact points, taking into consideration the difference in crown width between the premolars and molars.

Ideal arch coordination

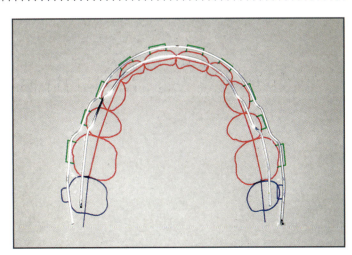

Fig 3-185 Coordinate the fabricated maxillary and mandibular ideal arches using the mandibular VTO produced before treatment. In this coordination, adjust in/out, offset, torque, and angulation, taking into consideration malocclusion that was present before treatment, referring to the pretreatment cast and intraoral photos. This is called *overcorrection*.

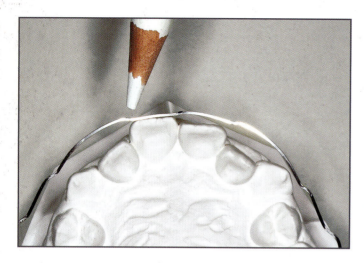

Fig 3-186 Considering the pretreatment state, offset (inset) and torque are added as overcorrection.

CHAPTER 4

Corrective Techniques:
Clinical Cases

Rotation of the Mandibular Anterior Teeth

Always consider the dental arch as a whole. Even in cases such as this one, in which a female patient aged 15 years, 9 months shows extreme rotation of an anterior tooth, it is not appropriate to consider correction of only one tooth. Such conditions should be evaluated as problems of discrepancy in the entire dental arch. Recently, a method in which the anterior teeth are simply reduced in contact areas then aligned has become popular, but this calls the basic purpose of orthodontic treatment into question.

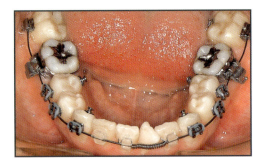

Fig 4-1a To obtain space at the mandibular right central incisor, an open coil spring is inserted between the central and lateral incisors (about 50 g, 2 months).

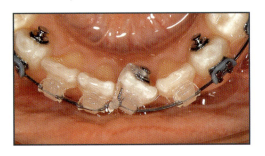

Fig 4-1b A lingual bracket is attached to the lingual side of the lateral incisor, and chain elastics are applied from the lingual bracket to the surgical hook applied distal to the central incisor. The memory wire (.016 × .016) is firmly placed in the slot of the right central incisor and ligated at a site mesial to the bracket (about 4 months).

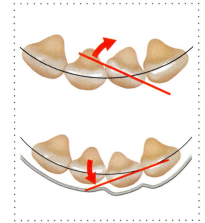

Fig 4-1d Overcorrection. The central incisor is mesially rotated *(top)*. Overcorrection is added to the ideal arch so that the central incisor is slightly rotated distally *(bottom)*.

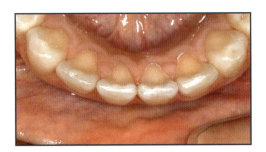

Fig 4-1c The ideal arch (.016 × .022 multiphase wire) is inserted and stabilized (about 4 months). When necessary, overcorrection is added.

Fig 4-1e After treatment. Proper tooth movement was achieved.

Rotation of the Mandibular Right Second Premolar

Be sure to consider anchorage. In this female patient aged 13 years, 4 months, there is space anterior and posterior to the second premolars due to congenitally missing teeth. In general, however, this space is often insufficient for the required movement. When the tooth is rotated around its axis from the buccolingual direction using an elastic, as in other tooth movement procedures, anchorage is important.

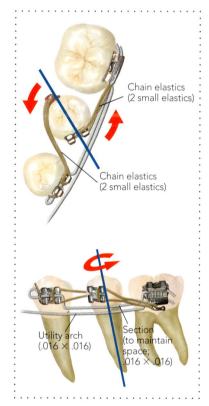

Chain elastics
(2 small elastics)

Chain elastics
(2 small elastics)

Utility arch
(.016 × .016)

Section
(to maintain space;
.016 × .016)

Fig 4-2c Rotation correction on the second premolar.

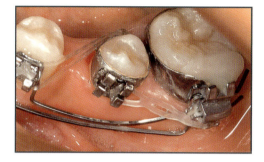

Fig 4-2a To improve the distal rotation on the second premolar, after banding or bonding, chain elastics are used. To maintain the space between the first premolar and the first molar, as well as anchorage, a section is inserted between the first premolar and first molar (.016 × .016 multiphase wire).

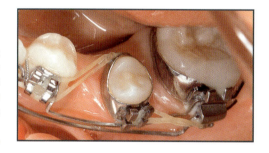

Fig 4-2b After 1 month, rotation has been corrected, but to compensate for possible relapse, the course is maintained for a few months until the tooth is in a slightly over-rotated state.

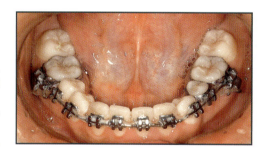

Fig 4-2d To prevent relapse, chain elastics are sometimes used after completion of alignment. (Ideal arch: .016 × .022 multiphase wire.)

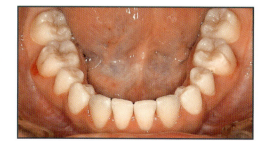

Fig 4-2e Immediately after removal of the appliance. To prevent relapse, the occlusal relationship, overcorrection, and design of the retainers are important.

Rotation of the Maxillary Central Incisors

Make a comprehensive diagnosis first. It is essential to make a complete treatment plan to correct discrepancy in both arches; do not focus only on rotating the maxillary incisors.

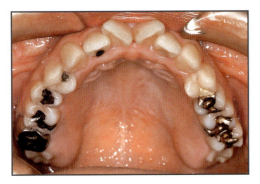

Fig 4-3a There is no space to rotate the central incisors in the maxilla of this 30-year-old female patient.

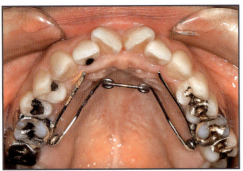

Fig 4-3b To ensure the space in the central incisor area and for distal rotation of the right and left first molars, a quad-helix appliance is applied (about 4 months).

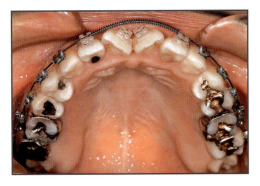

Fig 4-3c After lateral segment expansion using the quad-helix, further expansion is achieved using an open coil spring between the right and left lateral incisors (anterior segment expansion).

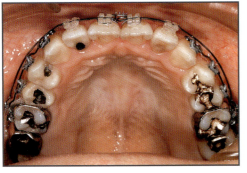

Fig 4-3d Alignment of the anterior teeth. After space was attained in the central incisor area using the open coil spring, the incisors were aligned using a utility arch with a T loop (anterior segment expansion). The T loop was distally rotated for overcorrection.

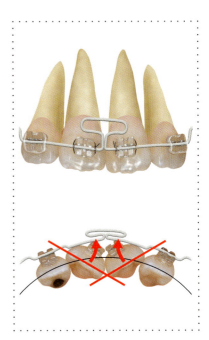

Fig 4-3e T loop.

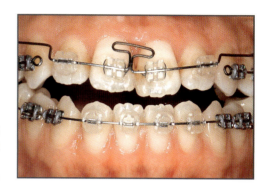

Fig 4-3f Overcorrection is added to the segment between the right and left incisors on the ideal arch.

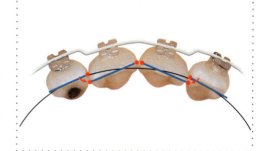

Fig 4-3g Overcorrection of the central incisors. The distal contact points of the central incisors are lingual to the mesial contact points of the lateral incisors.

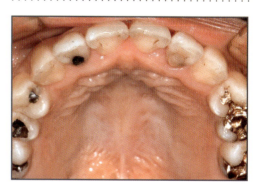

Fig 4-3h After treatment.

Correction of Ectopic Eruption of the Maxillary Canines

Consider the width and thickness of the alveolar bone and the direction of the tooth axes. The incidence of apically positioned canines is considerably high. The condition is sometimes similar to ectopic eruption. In such cases, attention should be paid to the width and thickness of the alveolar bone and the direction of the axis of the canines. Even when the crown of the canine is next to the central incisor, its movement is easy if the root is present distally and the axis tilts distally.

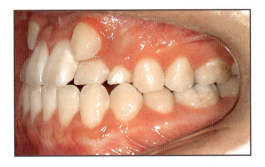

Fig 4-4a In this male patient aged 15 years, the maxillary canines are erupted immediately above the lateral incisors, and the primary canines are retained.

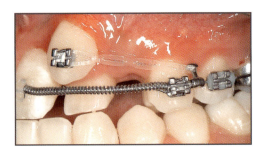

Fig 4-4b The primary canines are extracted. An open coil spring is inserted between the lateral incisor and canine; while the space is maintained, distal movement of the canine is attempted. A surgical hook is applied between the first and second premolars, and chain elastics are applied between the hook and the canine.

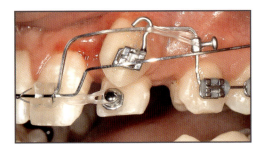

Fig 4-4c A large step is incorporated over the main archwire between the central incisor and the first premolar. A surgical hook is applied to the distal vertical leg, and chain elastics are applied between this hook and a hook placed on the canine to prevent distal tilting. Distal movement is continued.

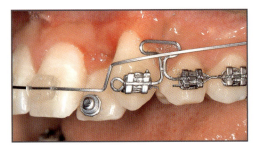

Fig 4-4d After completion of distal movement of the canine, a T loop is inserted to adjust the tooth axis.

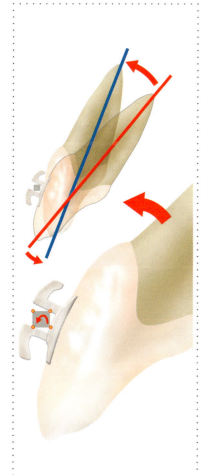

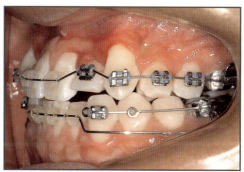

Fig 4-4e For labial movement of the lateral incisor, a memory arch is inserted.

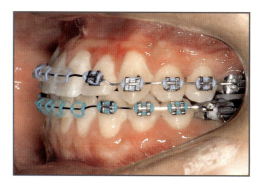

Fig 4-4f To correct the axis of the lateral incisor, labial root torque is added to the ideal arch (.016 × .022 wire).

Fig 4-4g Labial root torque is applied to the lateral incisor.

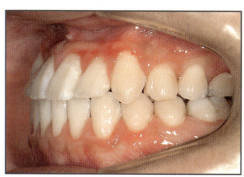

Fig 4-4h After treatment. Though the axis of the canine is good, the torque of the lateral incisor is less than ideal, partly due to the thickness of the alveolar bone.

Treatment of Lateral Open Bite

Determine the cause. When open bite of the lateral segment is observed, closure of the space alone is inadequate because the problem will recur if the cause is not addressed and corrected. This 19-year-old female patient had the habit of thrusting her tongue to the left during swallowing.

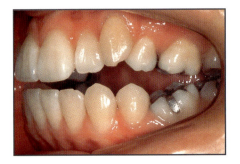

Fig 4-5a Open bite of the lateral segment due to tongue thrust and extreme mesial inclination of the mandibular first molar are observed. After resection of the lingual frenulum, tongue training and proprioceptive neuromuscular facilitation (PNF) were planned.

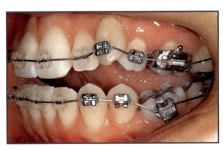

Fig 4-5b Memory arches are used for tooth alignment.

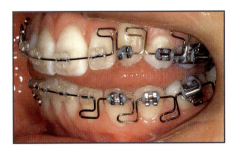

Fig 4-5c The mandibular first molar is uprighted using an arch with T loops (.016 × .016, heat-treated wire). For a certain period, tongue spikes are also used on the lingual side.

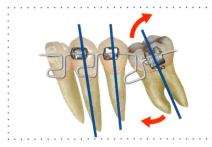

Fig 4-5d Labial root torque is applied to the first molar.

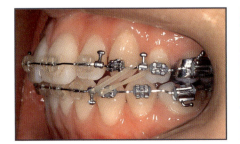

Fig 4-5e Class III elastics are applied between the maxillary and mandibular ideal arches.

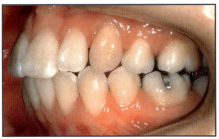

Fig 4-5f After treatment. The tongue habit and open bite are improved with myofunctional therapy (MFT), which is continued during the retention period.

Treatment of First Molar Crossbite

Crossbite may be a precursor to temporomandibular disorders. There are patients with first molar crossbite in the primary dentition who are not told of this condition during regular dental examinations. Crossbite may be a major factor in the subsequent development of functional impairment of the temporomandibular joint.

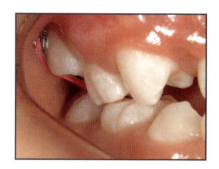

Fig 4-6a This female patient aged 7 years, 7 months presents with buccal tipping of the maxillary first molar. One lingual button is attached to the buccal side of the maxillary first molar and the other to the lingual side of the mandibular first molar.

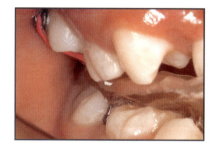

Fig 4-6b Application of a biotemplate to facilitate lingual movement of the maxillary first molar while preventing excessive extrusion and reducing pressure on the temporomandibular joint. Cross elastics are used with the biotemplate.

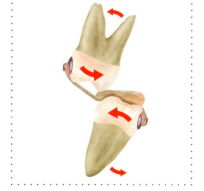

Fig 4-6c Correction of crossbite of the first molars using a biotemplate and cross elastics.

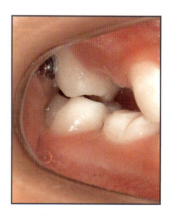

Fig 4-6d After 2 months, improvement of crossbite is observed.

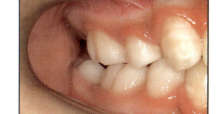

Fig 4-6e Completion of treatment.

Correction of a Step Between the Mandibular Second Premolar and First Molar

Steps must be corrected to attain dynamic equilibrium in function.

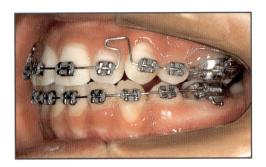

Fig 4-7a This female patient aged 9 years, 11 months presents with a step between the mandibular second premolar and first molar that has created a Class II canine relationship. When triple or double tubes are used for the molars, steps tend to develop; therefore, early correction is necessary.

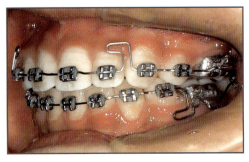

Fig 4-7b In the maxillary titanium molybdenum alloy (TMA) wire, a step-down bend is incorporated to a site mesial to the maxillary right first molar. In the mandibular wire, a step is incorporated in the L loop mesial to the first molar.

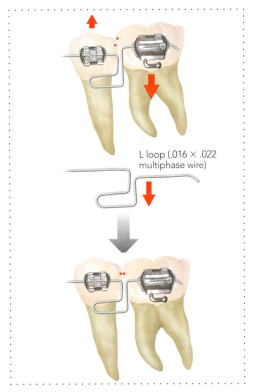

L loop (.016 × .022 multiphase wire)

Fig 4-7c Correction of the step between the mandibular second premolar and first molar.

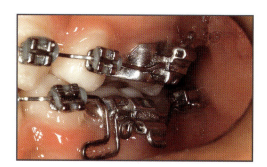

Fig 4-7d After 2 months, disappearance of the step and improvement of a Class II relationship of the lateral teeth are observed.

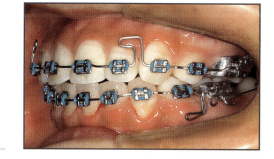

Fig 4-7e After treatment.

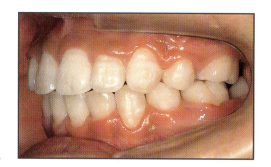

Fig 4-7f After removal of appliances.

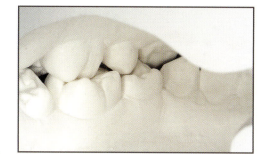

Fig 4-7g Lingual view of the occlusion on a cast made following treatment.

Correction of Class II, Division 2 Deep Bite in Adults

Consider the cause. As with open bite, deep bite cannot be corrected only by moving the teeth without identifying the cause of the problem. The mechanics are completely different depending upon whether the anterior segment needs to be intruded, the molar segment requires extrusion, or both are necessary.

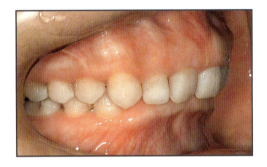

Fig 4-8a This 57-year-old woman's bite is deep in the anterior segment, and no mandibular anterior teeth are visible.

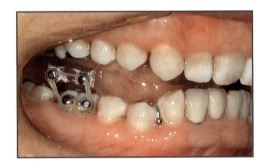

Fig 4-8b To correct the deep bite by extrusion of the mandibular left first molar, lingual buttons are attached to a biotemplate and the buccal side of the first molar, and an up-and-down elastic is used.

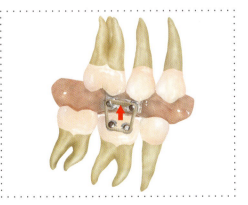

Fig 4-8c Extrusion of the mandibular first molar using a biotemplate and an up-and-down elastic.

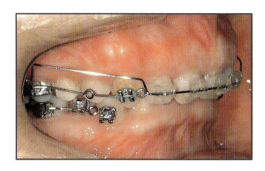

Fig 4-8d After 6 months, intrusion of the maxillary anterior teeth is begun. A stabilizing section (.0175 × .0175 TMA) is used between the maxillary canine and first molar, and a utility arch (.016 × .022) is used for the anterior teeth. A straight section and the utility arch are used for intrusion with torque application to the anterior segment.

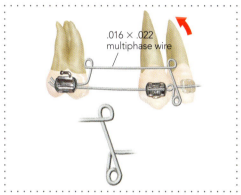

Fig 4-8e Lingual root torque is applied to the incisors using a torquing arch (.016 × .022).

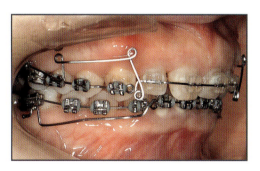

Fig 4-8f After 13 months. Since intrusion of the maxillary anterior teeth is advanced, a direct bonding system (DBS) is used on the mandibular anterior teeth for intrusion of these teeth as well.

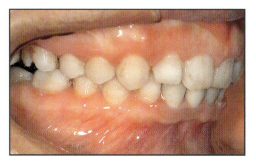

Fig 4-8g After 18 months. Completion of orthodontic treatment. Necessary restorative treatment can now be carried out.

Correction of Class II, Division 2 Deep Bite During the Growth Period

Growth and function are important considerations in the treatment of growing patients. Treatment methods for deep bite markedly differ for patients in the growth period compared with adult patients. After comprehensive diagnosis, treatment principles and mechanics considering the direction and stage of growth and function are necessary.

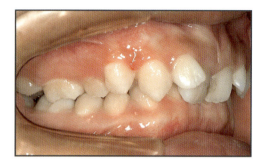

Fig 4-9a Extreme lingual inclination of the maxillary central incisors is observed in a female patient aged 14 years, 11 months. The bite is deep, and the mandibular teeth are completely hidden. As a result, the lateral incisors have a marked labial tilt.

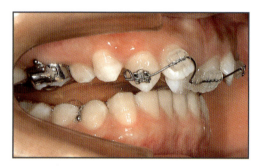

Fig 4-9b After 6 months. The most stable mandibular position is temporarily established using a biotemplate and PNF. Bands are used for the first molars and DBS between the canines. For alignment, a memory arch (.016 × .016) is used.

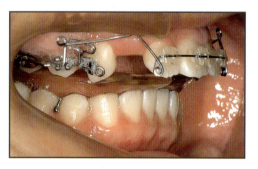

Fig 4-9c After 16 months. Both maxillary first premolars are extracted, and the canines are retracted (TMA wire). Contraction is performed while lingual root torque is applied (.016 × .022 multiphase wire). Note the amount of overjet after completion of distal movement of the canine. A biotemplate is used along with a contraction utility archwire (.016 × .022 multiphase wire).

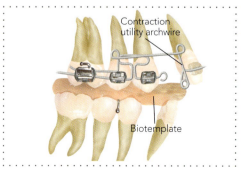

Fig 4-9d Contraction utility archwire and biotemplate.

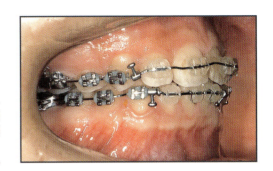

Fig 4-9e After 30 months. Torque and angulation of each tooth are adjusted, and the maxilla and mandible are coordinated (.016 × .022 multiphase wire).

Lingual crown torque

Esthetic bend

Fig 4-9f Torque and angulation are added to the ideal arch.

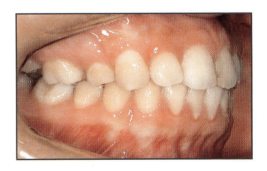

Fig 4-9g After completion of treatment. Note improved deep bite and torque.

Mandibular Dental Arch Expansion for Class II, Division 1 Occlusion

Pay attention to a low-set tongue. A narrow mandible may be caused by functional problems, particularly those related to a low-set tongue. The causes of a low-set tongue vary. In this case, a male patient aged 11 years, 8 months presented with shortening of the lingual frenulum. In addition, habitual function problems and the occlusal relationship with the maxilla are major factors. The appliances used to treat this case were specifically chosen to address these factors.

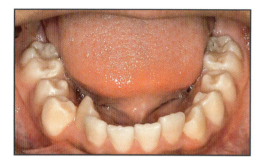

Fig 4-10a Linguoversion of the mandibular left canine and labioversion of the mandibular right canine are observed.

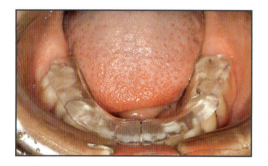

Fig 4-10b A biotemplate with a screw incorporated in the area between the central incisors is used for dental arch expansion. The screw is rotated once every 1 to 2 weeks.

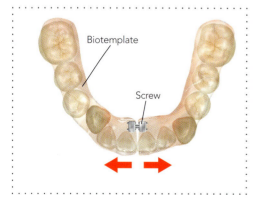

Fig 4-10c Dental arch expansion using a biotemplate featuring a screw.

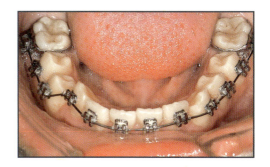

Fig 4-10d After 6 months, an expanded arch and a space between the central incisors are observed.

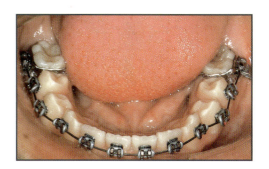

Fig 4-10e Bands and DBS, along with a memory arch, are used.

Fig 4-10f After 9 months, crowding in the area between the canines is almost fully corrected.

Finishing a Case in Class II, Division 1 Occlusion

Is marked overjet the only indication for finishing a case in Class II occlusion? In cases in which overjet cannot be corrected using a Class I molar relationship, so-called Class II finishing is sometimes performed. However, overjet may not be the only indication for using this approach.

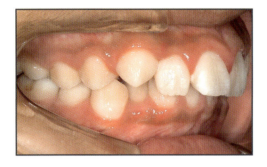

Fig 4-11a A male patient aged 11 years, 8 months presents with severe maxillary and mandibular crowding and marked overjet and overbite.

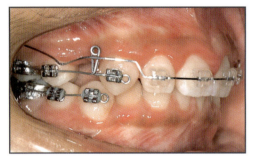

Fig 4-11b After extraction of the maxillary left first premolar, distal movement of the canine and intrusion of the anterior segment are performed. For the maxilla, a retraction section (TMA) and utility arch (.016 × .016) are used.

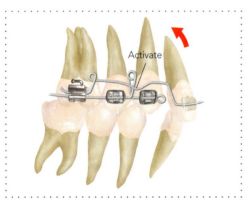

Fig 4-11c Correction of deep bite using a utility arch.

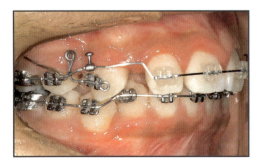

Fig 4-11d After 2 months. After successful intrusion of the maxillary anterior segment, DBS—along with a utility arch (.016 × .016)—is used for the mandibular anterior segment.

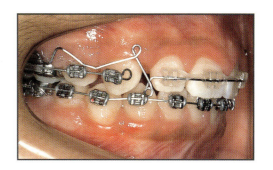

Fig 4-11e After 5 months. For lingual movement of the anterior segment, a contraction utility arch (.016 × .022 multiphase wire) is used.

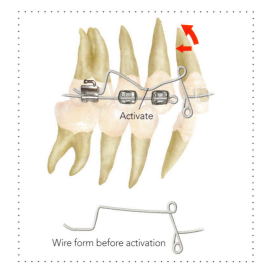

Fig 4-11f Contraction utility arch.

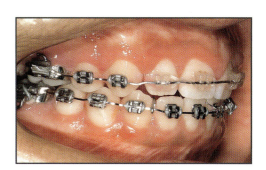

Fig 4-11g After 11 months. Adjustment of each tooth using maxillary and mandibular ideal arches and maxillary and mandibular alignment (.016 × .022 multiphase wire).

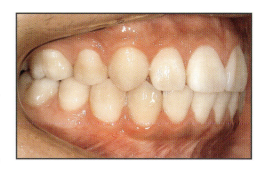

Fig 4-11h After 14 months. Completion of treatment. Not only crowding but also overjet and overbite are corrected. The molar relationship is Class II.